Psychosexual Medicine

PSYCHOSEXUAL MEDICINE SERIES

Edited by Ruth L. Skrine MB, ChB, MRCGP

Psychosexual Medicine is a discipline which uses a combined body and mind approach to problems related to sexuality, and which stresses the importance of the doctor–patient relationship. The method derives from psychoanalysis but is distinct in that the practitioner listens to unconscious material over a focused, narrow field. The work of many doctors and nurses and of some physiotherapists, provides opportunities for physical examination and treatment of the genital area which are unavailable to non-medical sexual therapists. Both physical and psychological problems and the interaction between them can be explored at the time of physical examination.

This series forms part of the developing body of knowledge held by members of the Institute of Psychosexual Medicine, formed in London in 1974. The books are for doctors and their colleagues who are interested in a psychosomatic approach to sexual problems, particularly those working in general practice and gynaecology, as well as psychological and genito-urinary medicine.

Other titles in this series

Psychosexual Training and the Doctor/Patient Relationship
Edited by R. L. Skrine

Introduction to Psychosexual Medicine
Edited by R. L. Skrine

Sexual Abuse and the Primary Care Doctor
Gill Wakley

Insights into Troubled Sexuality
Prudence Tunnadine

Psychosexual Medicine
A study of underlying themes

Edited by
ROSEMARIE LINCOLN
SCMO Family Planning and Psychosexual Medicine
Norwich Health Authority

CHAPMAN & HALL
London · New York · Tokyo · Melbourne · Madras

Published by Chapman & Hall, 2–6 Boundary Row, London SE1 8HN

Chapman & Hall, 2–6 Boundary Row, London SE1 8HN, UK

Chapman & Hall, 29 West 35th Street, New York, NY10001, USA

Chapman & Hall Japan, Thomson Publishing Japan, Hirakawacho Nemoto Building, 7F, 1-7-11 Hirakawa-cho, Chiyoda-ku, Tokyo 102, Japan

Chapman & Hall Australia, Thomas Nelson Australia, 102 Dodds Street, South Melbourne, Victoria 3205, Australia

Chapman & Hall India, R. Seshadri, 32 Second Main Road, CIT East, Madras 600 035, India

First edition 1992

© 1992. Chapman & Hall

Phototypeset in 10/12 Times by Intype, London

Printed and bound in Great Britain by Hartnolls Ltd, Bodmin, Cornwall

ISBN 0 412 43570 5

A catalogue record for this book is available from the British Library

Library of Congress Cataloging-in-Publication data available

Contents

Contributors

Peter Barrett MB BS, Mem. Inst. Psychosexual Medicine, general practitioner, Nottingham

H. Morag Bramley MA MB ChB, Mem. Inst. Psychosexual Medicine, specialist in genito-urinary medicine, Sheffield

Elphis Christopher MB BS DRCOG DCH, Mem. Inst. Psychosexual Medicine, senior clinical medical officer family planning and psychosexual medicine, London

Joan Coombs MB ChB, Mem. Inst. Psychosexual Medicine, honorary lecturer in psychosomatic gynaecology, Leeds

Katherine Draper, MA MB ChB, Mem. Inst. Psychosexual Medicine, senior clinical medical officer family planning and psychosexual medicine, Lewisham and Southwark, London

Mervin Glasser FRC Psych, consultant psychotherapist, Portman Clinic, London

Judy Gilley MB BS, Mem. Inst. Psychosexual Medicine, general practitioner and part-time senior lecturer in general practice, Royal Free Hospital, London

Gill Hinshelwood MB BS, Mem. Inst. Psychosexual Medicine, medical officer to the Medical Foundation for the Care of Victims of Torture

Rosemarie Lincoln MB BS, Mem. Inst. Psychosexual Medicine, senior clinical medical officer family planning and psychosexual medicine, Norwich

Tom Main MD FRCPsych DPM, Psychoanalyst, former president Inst. Psychosexual Medicine

A. Heather Montford MB BS DRCOG, Mem. Inst. Psychosexual Medicine, senior clinical medical officer family planning and psychosexual medicine, Queen Charlotte and Chelsea Hospitals, London

Ruth L. Skrine MB ChB MRCGP, Mem. Inst. Psychosexual Medicine, part-time senior lecturer family planning and psychosexual medicine, Bristol

Robina Thexton MB BS, Mem. Inst. Psychosexual Medicine, senior clinical medical officer family planning and psychosexual medicine, West London

Alexandra Tobart MB BS DCH, Mem. Inst. Psychosexual Medicine, former lecturer in psychosexual medicine, Nottingham

Gill Wakley MB ChB, Mem. Inst. Psychosexual Medicine, general practitioner, Staffordshire

Foreword

Elizabeth Forsythe

Doctors and nurses in family planning clinics, general practice, and in hospital out-patients, working in diverse fields including contraception, genito-urinary medicine, venereal diseases, gynaecology, or obstetrics may all be confronted with problems about sexuality. There is often a natural reaction of feeling at a loss, and a desire to look for an expert who can deal with such problems; but the patient has chosen this particular professional in whom to confide. This book is written for those who are in a position to receive such confidences.

While there are no experts in the field of sexual relationships, there are doctors and nurses who are prepared to listen, to be vulnerable, and to puzzle with the patient. Often, in telling his or her story to a receptive listener, the patient will be put in touch with his or her emotions, and thus be able to find a solution. The results can be surprising.

The traditional medical model of history-taking using questions and answers does not help, and can sometimes hinder understanding. As Peter Barrett writes in his piece on impotence, 'traditional training demands that doctors are knowledgeable, active, and in control. Psychosexual medicine is different. Each encounter with a patient is unique.' The need is for the telling of a story – the story of *this* unique person – and the telling can only be done in an atmosphere of trust and acceptance; hence the need for the professional to learn to listen. The man with impotence who frequently chooses to present his 'weakness' to a female doctor may do so because he has never had an opportunity to express his most intimate feelings without fear of being dismissed, rejected, or scorned.

The training provided by the Institute of Psychosexual Medicine and the contents of this book are about such professional listening. Examination of the genitalia is an opportunity not only for a special sort of professional intimacy, but can be the moment for the unveiling of many sorts of secrets, perhaps hidden even from the owner. The fantasies, fears, anger, and distress – possibly present for a lifetime – can be expressed, accepted, and looked at in *the light of present reality* with the help of the doctor or nurse.

The opportunity for replacing fantasy with reality is important, and Joan Coombs, in her sensitive chapter on problems with orgasm, writes, 'Much sexual activity that is depicted on television and in films and magazines involves the ultimate in sexual performance. . . real life is mundane and prosaic and for some the nearness to perfection is something that happens rarely.' The skill lies in being able to communicate a sense of reality while still honouring the patient's yearning for greater fulfilment through the sexual relationship.

This is not work for the expert who needs to feel powerful, the doctor or nurse who has the answers and can provide a cure. It is work for the professional person who is prepared to be vulnerable and powerless, who can be patient, courageous and sufficiently aware to explore the unique story with his or her patient – while resisting every temptation to instruct, treat, and organize.

Perhaps the work can be seen as a model for the understanding and treatment not only of psychosexual diseases, but of all diseases of the psyche and soma – that is psychosomatic disease – in a much broader sense. To quote from Morag Bramley's chapter on discharges and irritations in psychosexual medicine, '. . . sometimes the words used to describe physical sensations can be seen to be symbolic of the patient's feelings. Such words as "pain", "soreness", and "irritation" can apply to emotions as well as to bodily symptoms, and may provide a key to unspoken and often unrecognized emotional troubles. The doctor who can listen and think about the words used may be able to make sense of the situation. The emotion has probably been suppressed by the patient because acknowledgement would be too painful, and expression in the form of a physical symptom is easier.' Surely these words summarize much of the enigma of psychosomatic disease. The work can be an important and cost-effective contribution to preventive medicine, and can provide dramatic transformations not only in the health of the patient, but of the patient's relationships with his or her family, friends, and colleagues.

This book, written for the professional doctor and nurse, and for the interested lay reader covers much of the field of psychosexual medicine. Each chapter, written by a professional in the field, emphasizes the meaning behind the doctor or nurse/patient relationship, and how this can be used to help the patient's understanding. Psychosexual problems are approached via the symptoms that are most commonly presented – such as loss of interest in sex or impotence – and via a consideration of early and later development of sexuality in men and women. While problems in those of different ages are included, there is no upper age limit. The last chapter, written with profound insight and great wisdom by Judy Gilley on intimacy and terminal care, demonstrates that the psychosexual approach can shed light on the care of the whole person at any age.

1

Psychosexual skills and training

Ruth Skrine

SUMMARY

- Aetiological beliefs
- Presentation of psychosexual problems in primary care
- The doctor
- The psychosomatic genital examination
- The use of the doctor/patient relationship
- Method of study
- Training

In this book, the term 'psychosexual medicine' is used specifically to denote a combination of 'body-mind' doctoring. The form of medical practice described uses an interactional, dynamic method, which has its roots in psychoanalysis; at the same time, unlike most psychotherapies, it uses physical examination of the patient when appropriate. It can be seen as a specific form of psychosomatic, 'whole person' medicine. The work of a general practitioner requires him or her to consider every patient's problem in psycho-

Source: *Sexual and Marital Therapy*, Vol. 4, No. 1, pp. 47–58, 1989.

terms – weighing up the interaction between physical and nal factors at each consultation. Psychosexual medicine has more in common with this sort of doctoring than with sexual or marital therapy.

AETIOLOGICAL BELIEFS

The therapeutic orientation of any therapist will depend upon his belief about causation of sexual dysfunction. This belief is influenced not only by his individual personality, in that he will believe more easily the things that make sense to him, but also by the situation in which he works and the particular problems he meets. In over-simplified terms, this might mean that the psychoanalyst would see the causes of sexual problems as deeply rooted in infancy and earliest childhood; the behaviourist would consider previous learning experiences; and the marriage guidance counsellor would search for causes in the relationship between the partners. Psychosexual doctors firmly believe that unconscious factors interfere with sexual happiness, but that patients often express their unconscious tensions as physical symptoms and worries about the body. Of course, none of these belief systems is exclusive, and all of these factors are important, the difference in therapeutic approach being mainly one of emphasis.

The aetiological beliefs of psychosexual medicine have grown from the experience of doctors trying to help patients who have come to them for help. Thus the patients are a self-selected group, and may differ from those who would choose to go, for instance, for marriage guidance or counselling.

PRESENTATION OF PSYCHOSEXUAL PROBLEMS IN PRIMARY CARE

When a patient goes to a doctor he has certain hopes and expectations. One is that the doctor will be interested in, indeed may even examine, his body. He may also hope the doctor has some interest in his feelings. The majority of patients, although by no means all, consult the doctor independently, thus choosing a one-to-one relationship.

Masters and Johnson (1970) stated that 'therapeutic techniques emphasizing a one-to-one patient therapist relationship, effective in treatment of many other psychopathological entities, is grossly handicapped when dealing specifically with male and female inadequacy . . . the sexual partner ultimately is the crucial factor.' Many doctors working in a primary care setting would refute such a generalized statement. It has been found that an effective way of working, which is economical in time, is to treat the person who presents. If this is an individual by himself, then the doctor has the opportunity to focus on the doctor/patient relationship, which develops between him and that person. A patient who chooses to come alone may sense there are things inside himself, whether physical or emotional, which he would like to talk about. If a couple come together, it is best to see them together, at least in the first instance. The focus of treatment is then different, being on the relationship between the couple and their interaction in the presence of the doctor rather than on the one-to-one relationship of patient and doctor.

Those working in a primary care setting know that many patients only reveal a problem during a consultation for something else. Indeed, there may have been no conscious decision to discuss a difficulty, but patients may suddenly begin to cry, to say something unexpectedly, or just drop hints they hope their doctor will pick up.

Courtenay (1976) analyzed 100 consecutive cases of sexual disorder seen in general practice and found that only 18% complained directly. Forty-six percent has psychological symptoms, and 36% had physical symptoms, mainly related to the genitourinary system, the gut, or the skin. The range of physical and emotional complaints that can be associated with sexual problems, however, is much wider than might be suggested by Courtenay's figures. Table 1.1 (p. 14) shows a completely random selection, taken from a book published in 1987 (Skrine, 1987).

THE DOCTOR

Because so many requests for help hide behind other symptoms, the doctor has to develop particular skills in listening to the unspoken worries and complaints of his patients. The undergraduate training of doctors emphasizes the importance of taking a medical history, including a sexual history. It is the patient's feelings, however, about present and past events that are most important. If instead of taking a structured history the patient can be helped to tell their story in their own way, choosing the subject matter themselves, the important feelings are more likely to emerge.

Doctors often have more to unlearn than others in their efforts to listen to their patients. On the other hand, they are much more at home with the body, and can take less time than counsellors to find out what is happening sexually. Whereas counsellors seem to dance around exact details, doctors are much more direct, helped by patients who come expecting to talk and to be asked about their bodies.

General practitioners have a range of 'escape routes' they can use when things get difficult. As doctors we have a particularly wide choice of defensive actions, ranging from asking professional-sounding questions and giving prescriptions, to ordering tests and examining the patient physically. All of these may be appropriate for the doctor in some circumstances, but at other times they may be an escape from a difficult moment in the psychosexual consultation. Doctors can learn to stay with a difficult moment, think about it, and use it more fruitfully.

Doctors also are particularly practised in the doubtful art of reassurance. Of course, if the patient feels there are strong grounds to fear a physical disease despite exclusion by examinations and tests, that reassurance is appropriate and gladly accepted. Such reassurance, however, is useless when the basic anxieties have not been explored. Similarly, doctors are excellent at giving advice: but there are good reasons to believe that such advice does not work when the problem is related to people's private, complicated sexual lives. How easy it would be if people could be helped to enjoy sex by being told to do so!

It is clear, then, that doctors have special training needs that must be met if they are going to be able to listen to their patients, use reassurance carefully, and recognize that particular actions are sometimes a response to their own discomfort rather than based on good scientific principles. Psychosexual medicine, however, uses additional skills.

THE PSYCHOSOMATIC GENITAL EXAMINATION

The genital examination, used as a psychosomatic investigation, has little to do with teaching patients about their anatomy. It does have some use as a way of exploring body fantasies, perhaps particularly for women, and for both sexes it may reveal misconceptions about anatomy and function. The genital examination, however, is far more than this: it can be an opportunity for patients to get in touch with important feelings they did not know they had. It is worth remembering that the phrase 'the moment of truth', coined by psychosexual doctors, was taken from Hemingway's description in *The Sun Also Rises* of the moment the bullfighter *confronts himself* (Tunnadine, 1992).

> A middle-aged woman was already on the waiting list to see a gynaecologist about the deep vaginal pain she felt on intercourse. When she came for a cervical smear, the doctor asked about the pain. She said, 'Well, we don't do it much now because I don't feel like it.' The doctor asked how long this had been going on. 'About six months,' was her reply. 'What happened at that time?' asked the doctor. The patient burst into tears and said her father had died. The doctor provided paper tissues and they talked a bit about her father, how close she had been to him, and how she missed him. This took about ten minutes, and the doctor then took the smear. She found the uterus was leaning backwards, and was slightly tender when touched. She explained this to the patient, who confirmed that the pain she felt on intercourse was the same as that caused by the doctor's fingers.
>
> While the doctor did the paperwork the patient dressed behind a screen in the same room. Suddenly she said, 'Do you know, I think I've always had that pain, but I used to be able to wriggle about and make it all right. Now that I hurt all over, it's the last straw.'

It was perhaps unrealistic for this patient to expect to enjoy intercourse while she was still grieving so deeply for her father. The opportunity to share her grief with the doctor, who was also the person who examined her pelvic pain, seems to have been enough for her to put the two together by herself. Certainly she decided not to see the gynaecologist, and in due course when she came to terms with her father's death she was able to enjoy love-making again.

> A young woman complained to her doctor that she was unable to reach orgasm with her boyfriend. It was her

first sexual affair, and in the consultation she appeared quiet, shy, and rather withdrawn. She looked at the doctor with brief sideways glances only. Despite the apparent coyness, the doctor found herself calling her 'Mrs' by mistake, and sensed a hidden sexiness in the patient. Not much progress was made in the consultation until the patient said she wanted to stop the oral contraceptive pill and be fitted with a diaphragm. When she was lying on the couch she became quite giggly. The doctor, feeling her embarrassment but also sensing an underlying excitement, said, 'You seem to be fairly relaxed about this. Are you able to be like this with your boyfriend?' The patient clapped her hand over her mouth and said, 'Oh, I'm so afraid that if I really let myself go I will let out such a noise that I will make a fool of myself.' This opened the way to further talk about her need to be in control of herself and her fear of being 'silly'. She had not been very clever at school, and had felt she had to work hard at being sensible in order to gain her parent's approval. After two further consultations she was able to become orgasmic.

The vaginal examination provided an opportunity for the doctor to observe and to share with the patient a part of herself that had previously been hidden. During the two following consultations, the patient gradually showed more of the sexy side of herself to the doctor, both in her dress and in the content of their discussions. It seems likely that the rapid progress was due to the patient's opportunity to share the vulnerable, 'silly' bits of her body and her emotions with the same doctor who would continue to value her as a sensible person.

These two cases illustrate the importance of one person examining both the body and the emotions at the same time. The next case shows this also can be successful with men.

A couple came to the doctor because the wife had lost all interest in sex since extensive infertility investigations had shown them both to be subfertile. They wanted to adopt a baby, but felt this would not be right if their marriage was in jeopardy.

At the beginning of the interview the wife did most of the talking about her disappointment at not being able to get pregnant, and her attempts to drown this by working hard at her job. There was little eye contact between the couple, and the doctor had to try repeatedly to draw the husband into the consultation with remarks like, 'How did you feel about that?' Eventually the husband was able to say he was worried there might be something wrong with him because although his semen had been examined, no one had looked 'down there'. In response to this clear request the doctor offered to examine him, and asked if they minded if the wife stayed in the room. Both seemed happy with this, and the doctor and husband disappeared behind the screen, where his genitals were examined and found to be normal. The doctor noticed that the patient, while still lying on the couch, looked worried, so she said, 'They're fine, I can find nothing wrong. But you're looking worried.' At this the patient burst out his feelings about how awful the fertility investigations had been, how he had hated having to produce a specimen in the hospital toilet, and how vulnerable and exposed and angry he had felt walking down the corridors with his little bottles. After pulling up his trousers and coming out from behind the screen, his wife said, 'I didn't know you felt like that! Why didn't you tell me?' 'I didn't know myself how strongly I felt till now,' was the gruff reply. They started to talk between themselves, and by the next visit the wife was enjoying sex again. She felt that something inside herself had been punishing her husband for not feeling enough about their inability to have children. He, in turn, had felt he had to be 'strong' for her sake.

The important point in this case is that the genital examination – a vulnerable and exposed moment – allowed this man to get in touch with feelings he had not previously acknowledged to *himself*. It was fortuitous that his wife was there, and even if she had not been present he would probably have found a way of sharing his feelings once he realized he had them. As it was, most of the interpersonal work was done outside the consulting room.

Just a note of caution regarding this case: it is rarely useful for one person to observe the transactions between their partner and the doctor. Wherever possible, if two people are present the focus should be on the interaction between them.

These three cases demonstrate how very different emotions can be revealed during the genital examination: unresolved grief, a fear of being too sexy, and vulnerability mixed with anger. While a wide range of other feelings may be present, frequently neither the patient nor the doctor knows of these feelings or their nature until the moment they are expressed.

THE USE OF THE DOCTOR/PATIENT RELATIONSHIP

In common with many other professionals, the way in which psychosexual doctors use the therapeutic relationship has been derived from psychoanalytic theory. The work differs from other therapies, however, in that it uses a specific, focused approach to a small but important part of the patient's life. In contrast to the psychoanalyst, who listens to everything (Main, 1983), the doctor listens carefully to the patient's story but is trying to hear only a part of the unconscious material that is present. While listening and feeling with the patient, the doctor repeatedly 'pulls out' and thinks in particular about the 'here and now' in the doctor/patient relationship: What is this patient making me feel? Why am I acting in this way with this patient? What sort of atmosphere are we creating together? The way the patient treats the doctor and the reaction this produces in the doctor provides *living evidence* about that patient and his relationship with others. The doctor, while making allowances for his own professional strengths and weaknesses, can use the information gained from his feelings in an interpretation for the patient. All of this will be familiar to those who work psychodynamically with their patients.

Some patterns of interaction are gradually appearing in psychosexual medicine. For instance, the doctor who is trying to help a young woman to consummate her marriage may start by feeling protective and hopeful that she will be able to gently guide her young charge forward (even the not-so-young patients tend to be reported as 'girls' or 'lasses'). As time goes on, the doctor may become irritated and fed up. Neither the doctor/patient relationship nor the marriage is consummated; the patient manages to keep both the doctor and her partner out of her mind and body.

Or a man who has problems ejaculating in the vagina may inspire over-optimism in a woman doctor who is sure she will be the one who can help him, only to be frustrated in the same way his partner is frustrated.

Sometimes a doctor finds herself telling a woman all about female or male anatomy. If the doctor catches herself doing this, she may ask herself why this particular patient has not been able to gather information from all the sources available in our society. What internal inhibitions stop her 'hearing' what others have taken in so easily? It may be more productive to attend to that question than simply to supply more information.

The old-fashioned word 'frigid' can be an apt description of so many consultations in which the woman is unable to get in touch with her sexual feelings. The doctor who can recognize the interview itself as 'frigid' may be able to tolerate the cold, unyielding atmosphere more easily, changing from the questioning, probing attitude that is the natural reaction to such a patient to wait patiently for the first sign of a 'thaw'.

The therapeutic skill, however, does not lie in the recognition of patterns, but in studying each individual reaction *as it is happening* in the consultation and changing from minute to minute. Two brief moments from clinical encounters discussed in a seminar will help to illustrate this.

A patient of 25 years of age frequently visited her doctor complaining of indigestion. Tests did not show any serious physical cause, and the patient attended regularly for her 'white medicine'. One day she managed to tell her doctor that she had not yet consummated her marriage of five years, adding that she knew this was because she had been raped when she was 17 years old. She was referred first to a family planning clinic, where she 'didn't like the doctor', and then to a psychosexual clinic. There, she sat with her body, head, and eyes turned away, answering the probing questions from a doctor who usually listens well in monosyllables. The doctor became increasingly frustrated. 'Perhaps I should examine you,' she said. 'I don't let doctors touch me,' was the reply. The doctor, who felt that nothing she could ever do for this patient would be right, managed to say, 'I feel as if I'm treading on hot bricks, and anything I say will be wrong.' For the first time the patient looked up and said with venom, 'I don't talk to people I don't know.' 'Just as you didn't want to give yourself to a man you didn't know,' the doctor replied.

'He took something away that was mine, *mine*,' said the patient through clenched teeth.

The emotion shown at that moment was the first real contact between doctor and patient in what was to prove a stormy relationship. The patient's need to 'know' her doctor led to more questions about the doctor's private life than she was used to, but the recognition that the curiosity was an expression of the patient's particular problem made it easier to tolerate. The patient might have been particularly suitable for treatment by a trained general practitioner, as her need to know things about her doctor could have been more easily satisfied in a setting where the doctor was more accessible. On the other hand, such a relationship might have turned out to be 'too close for comfort' (Wakley, 1989).

The last case illustrates a moment in a series of consultations in which the doctor's awareness of her own feelings helped in the recognition that emotions being projected on to the absent partner came from within the patient herself (Main, 1966).

The patient was a cuddly, cheerful young woman who asked the doctor for help because she could not reach orgasm in the presence of a man, although she could do so by masturbation. She was relaxed and competent with the young son she brought with her, and talked to the doctor easily about her present happy marriage and two previous relationships. As she talked about her experience of the delivery of her child, however, the doctor perceived evidence of strong underlying emotions. The hospital routine was to mark the mother's reactions to her delivery on a four-point scale. The patient had been marked 'delighted' (point 3), but said, 'I knew I was "ecstatic" (point 4), but no one noticed.' The doctor felt apprehensive about the strength of her patient's feelings, and concluded that she must respond better than the hospital staff had done. However, she made no interpretation at that point, and encouraged the patient to go on talking.

The patient soon turned to her feelings during love-making, and how different and more exciting they were than masturbation. 'My husband wonders if he will be able to satisfy me by himself if I really enjoy it,' she said. The doctor began to speculate about this man in her mind, but then realized the remark could be a projection of the patient's own feelings. 'I wonder if you too are worried about the strength of what you might feel,' she replied. There was a long pause, and then the patient spoke of how frightened she was that she would enjoy love-making too much, and that it would take her over 'like a drug'. In the next session the patient talked about occasions in her life when strong emotions had led her into dangerous situations, and how her mother had not believed in her daredevil exploits.

The advantage of having only one patient at that time was that the doctor could deal with remarks in the context of the patient who made them. It is possible that the husband had his own feelings of inadequacy, but if the doctor had known this her attention would have been distracted from the urgent problem of this patient's fear of her own feelings. The doctor had been alerted to this by listening to her own fears and feelings of inadequacy caused by the patient. Perhaps the husband's feelings of inadequacy were evoked by the patient's fears in the same way?

METHOD OF STUDY

Case histories have been used to demonstrate the work of psychosexual medicine, and some attempt has been made to assess psychosexual work in numerical terms (Mears, 1978; Bramley *et al.*, 1981). This may not be a valid way to study and compare our work, not least because the patients seen in different settings are so different. Would it ever be possible to match genuinely two groups when the experiences of individuals are so different, and when the meaning of those experiences for each person is unique? Balint (1961) has said, 'To match patients according to age, sex, and social status is sadly insufficient, in view of the many further determining factors such as the occurrence and timing of deprivations in early childhood, the patient's attitude to authority, his sexual maturity and his ability to obtain regular sexual satisfaction.'

A good example of what can be done to express many years of careful clinical observation by reference to just four cases is given in the final chapter of this book. Also recommended is Marinker (1986) on the subject of narrative research.

TRAINING

Brown and Dryden (1985) and Cole and Dryden (1988) have discussed and described the training of marital and sex therapists. The training of psychosexual doctors differs substantially from all these methods.

The seminar method of training doctors was first described by Balint (1969). This method has been developed within the Institute of Psychosexual Medicine by training leaders who, although experienced psychosexual doctors, are not psychoanalysts. They in turn hold regular seminars for doctors, and also for nurses and other health care workers, such as physiotherapists.

The training is concerned with the acquisition of skills and does not include didactic teaching. It is important to understand that all trainees are fully qualified professional people taking total responsibility for their own work. They are not therefore coming for supervision of their work, or to obtain advice, but rather to have an opportunity to discuss particular examples of their work in detail. The emphasis is not on 'Was that right? Was that wrong?' but on, 'Why did that doctor act in that way with that patient?', and the crux of the matter, 'What light does that throw on the patient's problem?' Marinker (1987) refers to the particular atmosphere of professional seminars such as these.

Casement (1985), writing about the training of psychoanalysts, distinguishes the 'internalized supervisor' from the 'internal supervisor'. Although the approach of the seminar leader is bound to be internalized to some extent, the group training method encourages the development of an 'internal supervisor' from the beginning. The emphasis too is on 'learning from the patient' – the title of Casement's book – rather than on a theoretical framework into which the patient must be slotted.

Special emphasis, particularly during the training of leaders, is placed on the importance of training what has been called 'the professional ego' by not allowing individuals to reveal personal problems, or to allow the group to develop into a therapy group. This explicit distinction has not always been made in previous group training of doctors, and it is one of particular importance in the area of sexuality.

Basic training is fortnightly in term-time for at least two years. More than 1500 doctors have received such training since 1974, and the number of seminars throughout England has increased from nine in 1982 to 27 in 1991.

After four or five years of seminar training a doctor may apply to become a full member of the Institute by appearing before the panel. Assessment takes a day, and consists of participation in a seminar as well as individual discussion with two panel members.

The aim of training is that the doctor should show:

1. ability to understand the genital examination as a psychosomatic event, and to use these findings therapeutically;
2. ability to understand the contribution of both doctor and patient to the doctor/patient relationship;
3. sensitivity to unconscious elements in the patient's communications;
4. perception of the doctor's own individual strengths and weaknesses as a clinician;
5. ability to select cases appropriate to this approach, and to recognize unsuitable cases, such as those with deep-seated pathology or personality disorders, and those who cannot use interpretive therapy.

Criteria for accreditation of group leaders have also been evolved by the Institute of Psychosexual Medicine, and amongst other skills, leaders should be able to:

1. provide a model of human behaviour within a group by listening, understanding and meaningful intervention, aimed at freeing the members to perceive and express their own insights;
2. know the difference between a training and a therapeutic group and to confine group discussion to the needs of the former;
3. recognize factors which prevent the group from working and to free and enable the group to work again;
4. attend to the following: how does the patient being reported conduct their life and deal with the reporting doctor; how does the reporting doctor deal with the patient; how does the group respond to doctor and patient; how does the reporting doctor relate to the leader and the rest of the group; how does the group relate to the leader;
5. recognize group excitement and depression, collusive flight and distress and understand how these are related to the clinical material; the strengths, weaknesses and blind spots of individual members must be assessed and the leader must develop skill in focusing the groups awareness on the doctor/patient relationship.

Primary care workers meet patients with a great variety of sexual and psychosexual problems, which they will try to treat or relieve to the best of their ability.

The postgraduate training that is available to doctors and others includes courses in marital and sexual therapy. To these must be added those in psychosexual medicine, the particular nature of which has been outlined here. The doctor's choice will be influenced by his personality, his preferred way of working with patients, and the availability of training courses in his area. Further information about psychosexual training by the Institute of Psychosexual Medicine, the Prospectus and Bibliography are available from:

> 11, Chandos Street,
> Cavendish Square,
> London W1M 9DE,
> England

TABLE 1.1 PSYCHOSEXUAL PROBLEMS AND PRESENTING SYMPTOMS (Skrine, 1987)

There are many ways of classifying psychosexual difficulties, all of which are open to criticism. The following is not intended as a formal classification.

Presenting symptoms
  Pain on intercourse
  – with fiancée but not lover;
  – associated with female circumcision;
  – with history of incest;
  – and frequency of micturition.
Vaginal discharge
Pain during vaginal examination
Penile rash
Heavy periods
Abdominal pain and spastic colon
Breathlessness
Red eye
Depression

Table 1 Psychosexual problems and presenting symptoms 15

Presenting as a prescription request
To calm husband down.
For tranquilizers.
To dry up breast milk.

Presenting in relation to fertility control
Request for contraceptive pill
Problem revealed when collecting sheaths
Change of contraceptive method
Abortion request
Problem revealed during vasectomy counselling
Depression following sterilization

Overt psychosexual complaint
Impotence
Premature ejaculation
 − associated with sub-fertility
Non-consummation
Sexual dissatisfaction in women, including loss of interest
and lack of orgasm
 − following treatment of cervical erosion;
 − since marriage;
 − following birth of a baby;
 − since death of a baby.

Other
Psychosexual problem associated with terminal cancer.
Mother bringing daughter for check-up following rape.
Wife worried about husband masturbating.
Husband complaining wife is not interested in sex.
Patient asking doctor to show her where her clitoris is.
Patient refusing vaginal examination.
Woman worried because her boyfriend wants to live as a homosexual.
Patient complaining her husband makes unreasonable sexual demands.
Man of 60 complaining he is under-sexed.

Thirty-three patients presented in general practice, fourteen in family planning clinics, and one in each of the following settings: youth advisory clinic, vasectomy counselling clinic, hospital abortion counselling clinic, well baby clinic.

16   *Psychosexual skills and training*

REFERENCES

16
Balint, M. (1961) The other part of the medicine. *Lancet*, 7 Jan., 40–2.
Balint, M. (1969) The structure of training-cum-research seminars. *J. Roy. Coll. Gen. Prac.*, 17, 201–11.
Bramley, H. M., Brown, J., Draper, K. C. and Kilvington, J. (1981) Brief psychosomatic therapy for consummation of marriage. *Br. J. Obs. Gynae.*, 88, 819–24.
Brown, P. and Dryden, W. (1985) Issues in the training of marital therapists and issues in the training of sex therapists, in *Marital Therapy in Britain*, Vol. II, Harper & Row, London, pp. 301–37.
Casement, P. (1985) *On Learning from the Patient*, Tavistock Publications, London.
Cole, M. and Dryden, W. (1988) *Sex Therapy in Britain*, Open University Press, Milton Keynes.
Courtenay, M. J. F. (1976) Presentation of sexual problems in general practice. *Br. J. Fam. Plan.*, 2(2), 38–9.
Main, T. (1966) Mutual projection in marriage. *Comp. Psych.*, 7 (5), 432–49.
Main, T. (1983) The institute and psychoanalysis: debt, differentiation and development, in *The Practice of Psychosexual Medicine* (Ed. K. Draper), John Libbey, London, pp. 63–71.
Marinker, M. (1986) Workshop in research and communication. Inst. Psych. Med. newsletter, 7–15 Nov. 1986. (Limited circulation available from the Institute.)
Marinker, M. (1987) *Forward to Psychosexual Training and the Doctor/Patient Relationship* (Ed. R. Skrine), Chapman & Hall, London.
Masters, W. H. and Johnson, V. (1970) *Human Sexual Inadequacy*, Churchill Livingstone, London.
Mears, E. (1978) Sexual problems clinics: an assessment of the work of 26 doctors trained by the Institute of Psychosexual Medicine. *Pub. Hlth Lond.*, 92, 218–23.
Skrine, R. (Ed.) (1987) Appendix, *Psychosexual Training and the Doctor/Patient Relationship*. Chapman & Hall, London, pp. 388–9.
Tunnadine, P. (1992) *Insights into Troubled Sexuality*, Chapman & Hall, London (in press).
Wakley, G. (1989) The general practitioner as psychosexual doctor, in *Introduction to Psychosexual Medicine* (Ed. R. Skrine), Chapman & Hall, London.

2

The management of impotence in general practice

Gill Wakley

SUMMARY

- What can I do for you?
- Primary care treatment
- Referral for specialist help

Impotence in the medical sense is defined as 'erectile inadequacy'. In non-medical dictionaries it is defined by words and phrases such as 'powerless', 'helpless', 'decrepit', 'lacking in sexual power', 'unable to copulate, reach orgasm, or procreate'. No wonder people feel so awful about it!

WHAT CAN I DO FOR YOU?

Sexual problems are never easy for the patient to talk about or for the doctor to hear. It makes life a little easier for the doctor if the patient complains overtly: the young man who is worried he may be homosexual because he could not get an erection with a girl he fancied; the busy executive who is concerned that he

cannot satisfy his wife like he used to; the man with the menopausal wife who wonders if men have a menopause too, as he
cannot now 'get it up'; the divorced or widowed man who has
remarried or found a new girlfriend and wonders if he is 'too old
for that sort of thing' – all of these patients are able to approach
the problem directly, and all give the doctor something specific
with which to work.

Covert problems are more difficult: a man may ask if his blood
pressure tablets can be changed to the ones his friend is on;
another appears to have come to have a philosophical discussion
about his mid-life crisis; other patients ask for a check-up, or
complain of being tired all the time.

How do doctors faced with such requests find out if there is an
underlying sexual problem? Sometimes asking directly about sex
is the key, but the doctor may then gain the reputation of being
'only interested in one thing', which can frighten patients off. It
is only by constantly asking 'How is this patient behaving with
the doctor?', and 'What does this behaviour mean?' that the
doctor can hope to unravel the problem. For example, the patient
who makes the doctor feel impotent and helpless may be giving
a clue to an underlying problem of impotence.

Impotence means different things to different people. Lack of
desire or failure of ejaculation may be confused with erectile
inadequacy. Less commonly, premature ejaculation, or lack of
understanding of the refractory period after ejaculation may be
presented as impotence. Sometimes the erectile problem can be
a presentation of the partner's problem. Vaginismus, either primary, or secondary to infection or post-menopausal atrophy, may
be manifested in this way. Confusion can be avoided by listening
carefully to the story told by the patient and by not jumping to
conclusions too early; careful attention may reveal several possible
causes for the problem. Although each patient has his own particular set of problems, it is helpful to bear in mind some common
underlying causes, knowing that several could co-exist in each
patient.

Worries about performance with fear of failure are common.
Anxiety inhibits erection and will perpetuate any previous failure.
New relationships or restarting a relationship after a change, such
as illness, childbirth, or disability are frequent triggers. Concern
about the contraceptive method, or lack of it, is an effective
inhibitor of sexual function in both sexes. Fears and fantasies
about the genitals, or about the effect on them of masturbation,

disease, or ageing can be revealed. Drugs and illness can act directly on the physical process of erection, or can give rise to anxieties and fantasies, which then cause psychogenic impotence. Relationship difficulties, which may become obvious in the doctor/ patient interaction, may have been totally ignored by the patient, as the following case shows.

Mr F went to his GP initially asking about the dangers of conception for his 42-year-old wife. During this enquiry, he revealed he was having problems with his erection. As he told his story, the doctor began to feel anger about the way Mr F had been treated by his wife. This was his first marriage; he wanted a child. Mrs F already had an 18-year-old daughter, and Mr F and his wife had fallen out over her after he had caught the daughter having sex with her boyfriend in his house. Mrs F said it was nothing to do with him, but Mr F felt he wasn't having that going on in his own home. After the problem with his stepdaughter, Mr F had had an affair, but that was all over now and he was back with his wife. He wasn't even sure whether his wife had had her coil removed, although she had said she would. By this time the doctor was angry with Mr F as well! Recognizing his anger, the doctor was able to use this to show Mr F his anger with his wife and with the sexy teenagers, as well as his wife's anger at his behaviour. Bringing these things into the open helped his potency.

The shyness and embarrassment that may make it difficult for a man to complain openly about a sexual problem may also make it difficult for him to complain to his regular doctor whom he knows well and on whom he relies for his other medical care. For this reason it is often the trainee, new partner, or locum who is faced with such complaints.

Mr J breezed in looking purposeful and handed the locum doctor a long, white, quality envelope. 'I've been off to see a specialist – his report's in there.' He nodded at the envelope. 'He tells me there's nothing wrong physically with my wedding tackle, and said I should talk to my own doctor about it.' There was a short silence while the doctor read the letter, thinking to himself, 'This man has been off to see a specialist who is a stranger, and has now come to see another stranger.' He said, 'You must be finding this a difficult problem to talk about. Can you tell me a bit more about it?' There was a short silence before Mr J said, 'Well, it's like this. . .' He looked down at his feet and continued, 'I just can't seem to get it to work anymore. . .' Eventually Mr J managed to explain that he rarely had an erection nowadays, and had not had intercourse with his wife for 9 weeks. He hastened to say that she was 'very good about it', but he was increasingly reluctant to approach her in case it failed again. As the story unfolded, he became more fluent. The last time it had been all right was on holiday, when it had been 'most nights, no bother'. The doctor commented on Mr J's pleasure at that. Mr J replied that he had thought his problems were over, but it started again once they were home. Now he thought about it the situation had been much the same for some time, and worse recently since his promotion and now that he had even more work to bring home. The doctor commented on Mr J's brisk presentation of his problems, and how difficult he must have found failing at something so important when he seemed to be doing so well at work. The rest of the brief consultation was taken up with Mr J's attempts to look at how he felt about his work, how it impinged on his leisure time, and how inadequate he felt at not being able to control his work load.

Mr J demonstrated several precipitating factors: a change of job with more responsibility, physical tiredness, a loss in confidence in his ability to control his work, shame at his loss of potency, anxiety over his performance, and frustration and anger over the situation. The lack of communication of his difficulties, and his fear of ridicule from his regular doctor, had perpetuated the problem.

PRIMARY CARE TREATMENT

The doctor in a consultation, as described above, may end up feeling rather dissatisfied: he may never see the patient again, and may have no way of finding out if the patient was able to use the help he had offered. However, for many patients whose impotence is of short duration, resolution is rapid. Elucidation of the causes can in itself be therapeutic, as the patients can then find the remedies for themselves. Using the doctor/patient relationship during the story-telling and the examination can sort out the causes as the consultation progresses. Modification of the feelings of the patient takes place simultaneously with the diagnostic process. This clearly is a very different technique from the traditional medical model of a history of questions and answers followed by treatment as prescribed from on high. However, traditional questions do have a place in the management of impotence.

Traditional doctoring
The reasons for the patient's problem may become evident during the telling of the story. However, the patient may not realize the significance of some causative factors and omit them from his account, in which case some questioning to exclude these factors may become necessary. Specific questions about cardiovascular or neurological symptoms and drug treatment or misuse may be relevant. Drugs such as metoclopramide, cimetidine, anti-hypertensive medications and diuretics may be implicated directly, but some conditions for which drugs are prescribed are associated with increased sexual difficulties, such as depression or cardiovascular disease. Being labelled 'ill' may also cause sexual problems, either because of fear of the physical exertion involved, or as part of the powerlessness and vulnerability that such a label implies.

Baring the problem
As with other sexual problems, examination of the genital area is an important part of the diagnostic process in impotence, and may yield some surprising information.

> Mr S was a large, burly man with a slightly overpowering attitude. He was fairly well known to the doctor, having consulted her with excessive anxiety about many symptoms in the past. Now he wanted to know if he could catch thrush from his wife. No, he did not have any rash, soreness, or discharge. The doctor felt irritated, and, unwisely, without knowing yet what the problem was, leapt into 'Let's have a look at it then!' The doctor felt uneasy at the alacrity with which Mr S stripped off his trousers and pants and stood before

her. The ensuing erection demonstrated the absolute normality of the organ, and she was able to comment, 'An erection to be proud of!', thus acknowledging the sexuality of the moment. Mr S used this to tell her bitterly of his wife's constant complaints that he gave her thrush, and that recently his erection had failed several times when he had wanted to have intercourse. His wife saw his sexuality and his sexual organ as causing problems for her, and he had lost his erection.

Had he chosen to discuss his problem with his female doctor in the hope that she could value and appreciate his sexuality? This might explain the sexual feeling that made the doctor uncomfortable. However, she was able to say, 'So you came to the doctor to check it was all right,' thereby re-enforcing the 'doctor' image and banishing the vulnerable female one. The discomfort diminished, and the consultation was able to continue more easily.

Removal of clothing is often a removal of other barriers; defences are lowered and hidden problems revealed. Using the genital examination to explore the feelings of the patient about that part of his body, his fantasies, fears and expectations can sometimes lead to a quick resolution of the difficulty. Equally, a physical problem such as atrophic testes (a hormonal problem?); a cold penis with a diminished penile artery pulse (cardiovascular disease?); fibrotic plaques (Peyronies disease?); or loss of the cremasteric reflex (neurological disease?); may give pointers to further avenues for investigation.

Body and mind together
If the patient's story suggests that other physical examinations and investigations are indicated, they must be accompanied by constant attention to the doctor/patient relationship and to the patient's feelings throughout. It is no good cleverly elucidating that a patient has a physical problem with a pituitary adenoma without examining how the patient is feeling about having such an illness. Any chronic illness will cause difficulties with loss of self-confidence, possibly loss or changes in employment, anxieties about the future, worries about the family, and guilt and anger about the loss of previous good health – any of which may affect potency.

Mr H was a pleasant chap in his mid-30s who had had diabetes mellitus since his late teens. He was used to consulting doctors on equal terms about the management of his diabetes, and was able to broach the subject of his increasing difficulties with impotence with no apparent embarrassment. Throughout his account of his problems he remained remarkably unemotional, even dispassionate, as though it was happening to someone else. After some work on sorting out the various possible causes, it became apparent that he had quite severe diabetic effects with some kidney damage already, as well as hypertension and vascular disease. Any attempt to breach his defences and contact his feelings about this were in vain. At this stage he could only cope with the enormity of his future by shutting off his feelings. How much of his impotence was due to this emotional withdrawal and how much to his physical disorders could not be evaluated, nor did he wish to continue any work to find out.

Although several possible causes for impotence may become clear to the doctor, the patient may not be able to begin to deal with these at that particular time. Doctors are familiar with patients who, when first found to have a carcinoma, refuse all efforts at treatment, denying their illness and refusing to look at what the future holds. They need time to come to terms with the information. Similarly, the patient may refuse to accept the doctor's ideas about the causes of his impotence, especially when a mainly psychological reason is suggested. The patient may cling to the need for a physical explanation, and further screening for physical illness may be necessary, even where there is no indication from the history or examinations.

Screening would include hormonal investigations – free testosterone level, prolactin level, luteinizing and follicle stimulating hormone levels, as well as exclusion of other physical illness, with, for instance, haemoglobin and blood count, urinalysis, liver function tests, blood sugar, a full neurological examination, Doppler measurement of pulses, and so on. Occasional patients may be so afraid of losing their potency in other aspects of their lives that they cannot contemplate looking at any psychological factors until all physical avenues have been explored. These patients often demand specialist referral at an early stage of the investigation of the problem.

REFERRAL FOR SPECIALIST HELP

In an ideal world referral takes place after mutual agreement between patient and doctor for the purpose of obtaining a specialist opinion, or if the investigations or treatment are not available in general practice.

More commonly a hidden agenda provokes a referral after a decision either by the doctor, the patient, or the partner. This gives the specialist a complicated problem, and can prevent the referring doctor from having any further part in the treatment. Sometimes when referral is offered, especially if it is for 'potent' treatment such as injections, the patient may flee. If given a second chance – often possible in general practice – the doctor must start again and make a more accurate diagnosis. Flight from treatment is common where the patient has fears about potency or unconscious wishes to withdraw from sexual intimacy, or has been 'sent' by the partner to be 'put right'. If the general practitioner can sort out some of these problems, referral is more likely to be successful.

Mr B attended at the request of his wife, who had been accusing him of infidelity because of his lack of erections over the last six months, and was now threatening to leave. Mr and Mrs B ran a business together, and if she left it would be a financial disaster, so he had agreed to see the doctor to 'get it sorted out'. Mr B was charming but emotionally remote, and gave an impression of a man more interested in his work and the golf club than his wife: he worked all day with her and did not want to spend his social time with her as well. He thought they had just drifted apart but that she had not noticed. Mrs B had had a problem with her nerves and had had no time for him until recently. Now she wanted intercourse, and he 'couldn't oblige'.

Mr B agreed with every interpretation the doctor made, but shrugged his shoulders about making any changes. He was given another appointment to discuss things further but failed to turn up, although his wife did come. The patient here, of course, was the wife. She was the one complaining, not her husband who only attended to keep the peace. Mr B could only be helped if he accepted he had a problem and wished to change.

Before referral it is important for the patient to know and to choose the sort of specialist he would like to see. Some patients who have accepted that the problem is psychological will welcome an opportunity to explore their feelings with a psychosexual doctor; others want more detailed physical investigations and treatments such as injections. Some genito-urinary units that offer such treatments have a psychosexual doctor working within them, and occasionally such a doctor will provide a combined approach, as described in the next chapter.

The most satisfying referrals occur where specific specialist help is obtained while the interactions between the patient and primary care physician are continued and examined as treatment progresses.

Management of specific medical conditions is often thought of in terms of protocols or flow-charts. In the case of a symptom such as impotence, which has many different emotional and physical causes, 'management' needs to be much more patient-centred. The doctor has to follow the leads given by the patient by careful traditional doctoring and at the same time by being aware of the feelings generated by the patient in the doctor/patient relationship. The relative importance of the physical and emotional causes must be re-assessed at every stage.

3

Impotence: the referred patient

Peter Barrett

SUMMARY

- The referral and the patient's problem
- The doctor and the referral
- Papaverine in the treatment of psychogenic impotence
- Injections alone may not be enough

THE REFERRAL AND THE PATIENT'S PROBLEM

Why does the impotent patient ask to be referred? Superficially there is a wish to consult a specialist and not his own doctor about a sexual difficulty. However, this is not as simple as it appears. For example, the patient may lack confidence in the doctor's ability to help. The patient's past experience influences his perception of his doctor, and may have nothing to do with the actual capabilities of the doctor. The referring doctor will be left wondering what he has done wrong.

The patient can request a referral for more obscure reasons. If the relationship between doctor and patient is too friendly or too jolly, it may be difficult for the patient to disclose private, sensitive, and vulnerable feelings. The need to keep things 'social' in the surgery is a defence against the problematic emotional areas. Both doctor and patient may enquire after each other's family, pets, holidays, and a host of trivialities – anything rather than to face the sadness and distress of a sexual problem.

From the doctor's point of view, the interactions of referral are complex and two-way. Each participant has his own expectations and needs. Can the urgency of a referral be judged from the referring letter? The 'please see and treat' letter offers no clues. Does a full letter outlining the history and family background of the patient and his family provide any better indication? These details have already been filtered through one doctor/patient relationship and give an indication of what went on in that doctor's surgery. They cannot be relied upon to give much information about the patient's problem other than the study of that patient by that particular doctor. Often an urgent appointment is arranged by a GP for a patient 'in desperate need of help' and the patient does not turn up. Clearly something has gone wrong. Is it the GP who is in need of urgent relief from the patient's distress, rather than the patient? The need to be potent in dealing with an impotent man is strong. The patient might not be able to face looking at the problem, and finds some excuse not to come. The person referred may not actually be the patient, and demonstrates this by non-attendance. Or is the patient being powerfully impotent and showing his anger by 'not coming'?

A 50-year-old man was referred by his GP to the psycho-sexual clinic. The man bounced into the room and sat down, arms on the table, leaning across at the doctor. 'I expect "John" has written to you about my little problem' he said. 'I had a bit of a chat with him but we didn't get very far, and he suggested that I come and see you.' He seemed very chummy with his GP but it turned out his doctor believed in using first names with all his patients. The doctor went on to explore the nature of the sexual difficulties. It seemed the problems lay in the patient's tremendous anger with his wife, and after a 45-minute consultation the patient appeared very relieved, saying, 'I think I knew about my anger all along, but I just couldn't talk about it with my GP. I know him far too well.'

The pride the GP had in knowing and befriending his patient had interfered with the patient's ability to talk freely; the professionalism of the GP's consultation had been undermined by his need to be friendly.

The request for referral may be used by the impotent patient to maintain the *status quo*. He will obediently go along to the clinic, and after no improvement will proudly declare to his partner that nothing can be done. Impotence can be a powerful means of defeating both partner and doctors.

A 64-year-old man attended the clinic with his wife, who did most of the talking while casting damning glances at her husband when describing his limp and useless penis. The man sat quietly, looking to one side. Their mutual anger was almost palpable. The doctor asked the man what he felt about the situation. He said, 'I think it's my age, doctor. I don't think anything can be done about it.' The doctor continued the consultation, but realized he was doing most of the talking as the man was monosyllabic in his replies. It was suggested the man come back to talk on his own, which he seemed to agree to readily enough.

At the next session, he turned up on time, leaving his wife sitting in the waiting-room. The second session, however, was just a fruitless. The man was 'not giving' and not interested in thinking on any level about the problem – physically or emotionally. This was interpreted back to the patient, who said, 'I didn't think you could do anything,' and left. He had been successful both in rendering the doctor impotent to help, and in continuing to demonstrate his angry impotence to his wife.

THE DOCTOR AND THE REFERRAL

What of the patient's doctor? Why and when does he decide to refer? Who does he decide to refer? If the doctor chooses to refer the patient, is it because the patient wants to go, or is it because the doctor thinks it appropriate? The answers to these questions have a marked effect on the subsequent consultations.

Traditional medical training demands that doctors are knowledgeable, active, and in control. Psychosexual medicine is different. Each encounter with a patient is unique. The trained psychosexual doctor does not have a set of answers or treatments ready to hand. Each encounter is fresh, and the demand on the doctor is to concentrate on what is happening between the patient and him or herself in the consultation, and to use these observations to interpret the patient's behaviour. Many doctors are uncomfortable with this approach. Their worries about lack of knowledge and fears of opening 'a can of worms' often results in a precipitate referral to 'the specialist'.

Some doctors need to be active all the time. There is, without doubt, great satisfaction in treating a condition like myxoedema with thyroid hormone and observing the dramatic improvement. But what of the impotent man? After taking a history, doing an examination, taking bloods for liver function and testosterone levels and finding them all normal – what then? The sense of impotence in the doctor – his impotence to do anything more – is great. How does the doctor deal with this feeling? He can give injections of testosterone in the hope they will work, and sometimes, because of the placebo effect, they do work for a while. He can attempt to defuse the problem by reducing his patient's expectations, or those of the patient's partner; or perhaps trivialize the whole thing and hope it will just get better on its own. None of these solutions are likely to be helpful, and the doctor may then resort to referral.

PAPAVERINE IN THE TREATMENT OF PSYCHOGENIC IMPOTENCE

The use of papaverine injections is a recognized means of achieving erections, but it is not without its problems. The shift of emphasis from dealing with the whole patient to dealing just with the penis means that the entire procedure can become purely mechanical, resulting in no long-term benefit to the patient. However, if used carefully in conjunction with the skills of the psychosexual therapist, it can be a useful adjunct to the consultation.

The physical problems of giving papaverine are well documented, notably priapism and the occurrence of fibrosis at the injection site, meaning that the injections should only be given with full and informed patient consent.

The injections are given direct into the corpora cavernosa of the penis, and in a large number of cases result in an erection within five minutes. The fact that the penis is still in working order can relieve the patient's fear; it can also provide an opportunity to observe the patient's reaction to his erect penis.

A 30-year-old man was referred to the psychosexual clinic by his GP. He was a new patient at the practice, and gave an 18-month history of erectile failure. He no longer had morning erections and had lost his libido. His GP felt his problems were the result of back trouble, but a consultant had given him a thorough examination and found no abnormality.

The patient arrived at the clinic rather early for his appointment. He was a smartly dressed rather 'cocky' man, who had a very disdainful manner. He related much the same story as in the referral letter. Prior to one-and-a-half years ago he had been perfectly well apart from the occasional premature ejaculation. He described longish relationships with two girlfriends, but he was no good sexually with them and had returned to a previous girl who was much more understanding. Although he was happy with her, he did not see the relationship lasting long; he was not interested in long relationships. He told the story of his failures in a detached way with little emotion. Despite many attempts on the doctor's part to get him to look at his feelings, he was unable to do this. It was very unlikely that he would be able to make use of any psychotherapeutic technique.

The whole problem of impotency was focused on this man's penis, and there was little chance of progress until the focus could be shifted. The patient was quite unwilling to do this, as the thought of having to look at his feelings was too threatening. The doctor decided to introduce the possibility of injections of papaverine.

Having had a full explanation of the possible side-effects, the patient agreed to an injection and returned the following week. He was given a test dose of 10 mg of papaverine and responded well. His face showed evidence of his relief, and as he sat down after the injection he started opening up about his feelings. He had a very chauvinistic attitude towards women, and was always keen to protect and look after them. They seemed to him to be a different race. At the next session another injection was given with similar effect. Little by little he let his feelings out. His father was very old fashioned. His mother was protected by her husband and son, and they never rowed. He had learnt to deal with his feelings by getting them 'over and done with'. Women had to be pleased no matter what he really thought about them. Expressions of anger were not allowed, especially towards his mother. At the next session he reported he was much better, and had started to get spontaneous erections again. The doctor wondered whether the man's outwardly protective attitude towards women was really covering his anger and disdain. The patient said he had not realized how angry he was until then. It was suggested that he return in a fortnight's time. He arrived a little late, and reported that things were very much better. He seemed to be standing up for himself in all sorts of ways, even being late for his appointment. He did not think he needed to attend again.

Here, the use of papaverine allowed the patient to feel safe enough to start looking at his feelings. He needed to know that his penis was capable of functioning again before any shift in emphasis could occur. As well, the availability of an active physical treatment may have helped the doctor to feel less impotent in dealing with this difficult doctor/patient relationship, allowing breathing space for both patient and doctor.

If the practice of psychosexual medicine were a purely psychotherapeutic technique, this invasion by mechanical means would be unthinkable. But the skills of a trained doctor are applicable to a wide range of doctor/patient encounters. Here, it was not just a case of showing this man that his penis was 'normal' and then saying, 'Get on with it', but of understanding the nature of his fear and anger, and allowing him time and space to come to terms with it.

INJECTIONS ALONE MAY NOT BE ENOUGH

The emphasis on dealing with the whole person emotionally and physically, as is the norm in psychosexual medicine, can be jeopardized by the use of injections. Some doctors deal purely physically with impotence, with scant regard to the doctor/patient relationship. All the patient is left with in these circumstances is an erect penis!

> A 55-year-old man was referred by a consultant, having had a series of papaverine injections which had been 'very successful'. The patient had obtained good erections, and had been instructed on how to do his own injections at home. When he attended the psychosexual clinic, however, he looked very glum. He knew the injections were very good, and the consultant had been very patient and understanding. The only trouble was they were too mechanical: he could not bring himself to do them. He had made love once but could not do it again.
>
> In the presence of a doctor who was interested in other parts of his life as well as his penis, he began to talk about his children, of which he had three, two of whom still lived at home and were in business with him. He felt very protective of them, and made sure nothing went wrong when they were dealing with clients. Further exploration, however, revealed deep resentment, anger, and frustration at the fact that his sons were still at home. He felt he had no privacy, and they seemed to him to be usurping his position in the business. His wife was very loving, but stood up for her sons at home. The man was able to make use of the doctor's interpretations of his anger. He re-organized the business, set up a new one for himself to run, and started standing up for himself at home.

It was useless merely to give injections to this man. Although the penis was erect after the injection, he was not going to use it when he felt so angry and resentful with those around him.

The apparent efficacy of papaverine can blind the doctor to the interaction between him and the patient. It is easy to fall into the trap of traditional medicine and reassure the patient that all is well because there is a demonstrably normal erection. Just because the doctor knows the patient is normal does not mean the patient feels the same way.

> An 18-year-old man was referred because of his impotence. He had never been able to achieve satisfactory

intercourse, and described a series of failed relationships in a miserable, downcast way. Every time he came
to make love, his initial erection went down. For three
long sessions the patient and doctor struggled to reach
an understanding of the man's problems. The patient
seemed unable to expose his emotions; although there
was no physical reason for his impotence, there was no
way through his emotional barriers. The doctor suggested the use of papaverine injections, to which the
patient readily agreed, perhaps to avoid any further
emotional probing.

An injection of 15 mg of papaverine was given and
resulted in a splendid erection. The patient, however,
did not look quite so impressed. The doctor said, 'Well,
that seems to be working well. I wonder how it seems
to you?' The patient looked down and said, 'Oh, is it all
right? It doesn't seem very big to me.' The doctor was
able to use this to explore the patient's self-image. The
young man had never felt good enough for women, and
felt criticized and ridiculed by them. This led on to an
exploration of his earlier life, including a critical mother
and mocking girlfriends.

Without the use of papaverine it is doubtful whether this man
would have been able to progress. It was not, however, simply
the injection that produced results: the effects of the injection also
had been explored; he had not just been fobbed off with reassurance that his penis worked satisfactorily. It is all very well for the
doctor to know that the patient is all right; it is a very different
thing for the patient to know and to accept this for himself.

Papaverine does not work for every man. The puzzle is why,
in the absence of any physical abnormality, it does not.

A 68-year-old man of military bearing, wearing regimen-
tal badges, was referred because of impotence. He did
not achieve erections at any time, and had not done so
since the death of his wife. Since then he had hidden
himself away from all social contact, but eventually was
persuaded to go to a social club, where he had met a
'wonderful woman' who he believed had saved him
from suicide. The relationship had deepened, but when
they had tried to make love he had failed completely.
He felt devastated and wanted to break off the relation-

ship, but she wanted to continue. It was at her suggestion that he had sought help.

Some time was spent in the first interview determining whether it actually was he who wanted help. Eventually he decided he wanted help on his own behalf and not just to please his girlfriend. It was impossible to get near the emotional content of the problem. His defences were enormous, which was all that had been established by the end of the second session. The doctor raised the possibility of papaverine injections, and should have been warned by the reply: 'If you think it will help, doctor.' Gradually increasing doses of papaverine were given. After each injection there would be a half-hearted erection lasting a few minutes. The doctor was disappointed by the result but noticed that the patient did not seem to be as concerned. The doctor said, 'You know, in some ways you seem relieved about these injections not working. I wonder why that might be?' The patient sighed and was able to say that although his girlfriend was a wonderful woman, he did not think she could ever match up to his wife. The trouble was, he felt grateful to her and did not want to hurt her.

The doctor and the patient had played the game to its conclusion. Everything that could have been reasonably expected of him he had done; his girlfriend could not blame him for not trying, nor could he blame himself. The relationship was thankfully at an end. He returned to his memories of his wife. Not even papaverine was potent enough to overcome his emotions.

There is no doubt that the use of papaverine has widened the scope for doctors trained in psychosexual medicine if they feel comfortable using the technique. What seemed at first dangerous, limiting, and mechanical has not proved necessarily to be so. Patients must be warned about side-effects, and the injections only carried out with their full and informed consent. But if the reactions of the patient and the doctor to the injection are studied, then there are opportunities to make progress in cases which would otherwise founder.

Mention should be made of the various devices used to mechanically induce erections. They are designed to create a vacuum around the penis, so sucking blood into the organ. Once the penis is erect, a rubber ring is placed over the base of the penis to maintain the erection. Many patients do not wish to use these devices, believing them to be too mechanical.

In men with organic impotence who do not wish to use injections, or in those who have developed fibrosis as a result of papaverine, operations to replace the erectile tissue with implants of rubber have been successful. It is important to arrange counselling before the patient agrees to an operation. The dangers of focusing only on the patient's penis have already been described. It is crucial that before performing an irreversible procedure, every opportunity is given for discussion and exploration of the emotions. There is no excuse to avoid the patient's feelings about such a procedure just because there is a physical cause.

4

Ejaculatory difficulties

Robina Thexton

SUMMARY

- Premature ejaculation
- Cultural differences
- Being 'good enough'
- Behavioural or interpretive therapy?
- Non-ejaculation
- Self-motivation
- Reluctant fathers

Little boys enjoy having a penis and are proud of their erections from an early age. They become aware of the adults' attitude towards their interest in their genitals, and if this pleasure is frowned upon they may feel ashamed and become secretive. Nocturnal emissions begin at puberty, and although they may have occurred earlier, now the ejaculation becomes forceful. Competition between boys about the distance to which they can ejaculate is well known.

Ejaculation is a psychosomatic event, controlled by the autonomic system and by the cerebral cortex. Ejaculation of semen happens at the time of orgasm and, at its best, gives a sense of fulfilment and relaxation afterwards. The first experience can, however, frighten a boy because of the overwhelming sense of losing control.

Men consult their doctors if they have difficulty holding back ejaculation, so that orgasm occurs too quickly, or because ejaculation does not happen in the vagina during intercourse, or sometimes does not happen at all. Cases described here concern those problems which present during heterosexual relationships and are psychogenic in origin. The physical causes of ejaculatory problems have been well described elsewhere (Bancroft, 1989).

PREMATURE EJACULATION

This is a term used if the ejaculation occurs even before penetration, or so quickly afterwards that sexual pleasure is disturbed. A number of attempts at more precise definitions have been made, and include those based on the amount of time in the vagina following penetration (one-half to two minutes), to those depending on the ability of the woman to reach orgasm (Masters and Johnson, 1970). None of these is very satisfactory. It is interesting that a large study found that two out of three men would like to last longer (Kinsey *et al.*, 1948), and perhaps the reaction of the man to what is happening is the most important factor. He may feel deprived of full satisfaction by the prematurity, but often it is the woman whose pleasure is disturbed by the rapid ejaculation – orgasm is not possible and she feels frustrated and angry – and her reaction in turn is upsetting. In addition, she may play an unconscious role in her interactions with the man, which can contribute to his problems. Control of ejaculation can be seen to be concerned not only with the man getting control of himself, but of his feeling safe enough to gain this control in the presence of a woman. Such safety may be threatened by unconscious fears of the vagina, or fears about her power as a woman. The woman herself may in turn have her own inhibitions which make it difficult for her to respond, and allow him to take control.

Primary and secondary premature ejaculation

Premature ejaculation can be primary or secondary, and there are many causative factors of each. Primary premature ejaculation is the failure to control ejaculation with the sexual partner (it seldom occurs in masturbation), and is commonly due to anxiety and lack of sexual confidence. Young men tend to be easily excited and ejaculate quickly, and are often in situations where speed is necessary, as when they are likely to be disturbed. Secondary premature ejaculation occurs through stress due to financial worries, work or illness, a variety of drugs, and sometimes fear of pregnancy or worries about sexually transmitted diseases. Other well-known causes include bereavement, the impending break-up of a relationship, or guilt about a secret affair. Where the man's attitude toward himself as a sexual being has not fully matured there are other, less conscious, feelings that can cause anxiety. Commonly there is unconscious hostility towards women, which is a hangover from earlier relationships. Anger is a frightening emotion, especially to a child, and especially when the object of the anger is a close and loved person. At the time it is felt to be safer to suppress the anger, which can cause problems in later relationships.

The following case shows how, by the use of the here-and-now in the consultation, the doctor is able to help the patient to see how he shuts women out because he is angry that they do not seem to appreciate his needs.

A 35-year-old man requested an appointment at the clinic where his wife obtained her contraceptive pill. She had mentioned their sexual disappointment to the family planning nurse, who told her about the session for psychosexual difficulties. The man made his own appointment and arrived early. He said, 'Because I can't last long enough, we're both frustrated, and so we don't have sex much now.' He was a good-looking man, but had a rather distant manner as he talked about himself. He grew up in Scotland with a mother who was very strict and who frequently rebuked him for under-achiev-ing at school. He said she showed him no warmth. 'We have to ask her to stay with us so she can see her grandchildren, but I can't find anything to say to her.' He did not mention a father, but talked admiringly about his wife and her domestic and mothering skills. His blood pressure, urine test, and genital examination were all normal, and he did not show any anxieties about his penis. The doctor was puzzled, and in her wish to improve the situation said to the patient, 'I'll give you another appointment, and perhaps I can stumble upon some insight into why you have premature ejaculation. It will teach me something about this common problem.' Here the man erupted angrily, 'I'm not coming for you to get insight; I want some help for myself!' The doctor felt foolish, put-down, rejected, so she said, 'I feel really shut out by what you just said.' After a pause he said, 'That's what my wife says – she feels emotionally out in the cold with me.'

Suddenly the doctor pictured a small boy in Scotland, shutting himself off so he would not feel so hurt by his mother's strictness, and never being able to answer back. In the safety of the consultation the cork had come out of the bottle and he had shown his anger. Such an explosion of feeling can be compared to the uncontrolled letting go of orgasm and ejaculation. When the doctor said what she was feeling, the patient himself linked it to how his wife felt.

The doctor shared her recognition that he had not been able to give his wife enough because he believed women never appreciated his needs, and therefore he could give nothing in return. This allowed the patient to return again to his feelings that women always have the last word, and that in this respect his wife was like his mother. In her professional capacity the doctor did not need to compete with the patient for attention, and in the consultation the patient had the novel experience of being allowed the last word himself. He went home and was able to share some of his deeper feelings with his wife and the premature ejaculation improved.

He had two further consultations with the doctor to consolidate the work that had been done. In the presence of an older woman doctor he was reminded again of his mother, and talked further about keeping his feelings to himself in order to suppress his anger at being dominated. When last seen, he reported that he and his wife were both much happier with their sexual life.

The motivation of this patient to get help for himself was high. Although the first approach had been made by his wife, he had taken up the offer of help and had come by himself, clearly wanting to solve the problem. He was able to listen to the interpretation of the doctor/patient interaction, and to make changes in his attitudes.

Less success can be expected in the highly defended man who believes that only a pill or an injection can possibly cure him, and that the trouble is due to some local difficulty with the genitalia, or some deficiency of his hormones.

CULTURAL DIFFERENCES

An attractive Jamaican came to see the doctor with a complaint of premature ejaculation. He described his mother as being 'mouthy', meaning that she shouted a lot. He seemed to assume the doctor should cure him, which made her feel 'mouthy' too. He said his girlfriend was 'mouthy' and that he admired her for this, but could not control her or himself. She was by this time sleeping in another room. Despite doing the usual blood tests to prove the problem did not lie in his hormones, he still expected the doctor to produce a magic cure, and was quite unable to communicate on an emotional level, or to use any interpretations. After three visits he gained no insight into his problem, and failed to attend again.

When the patient and doctor are from different cultures, there can be additional difficulties in understanding the consultation. This may be due to subtle differences in the use of language, a problem that was present to some degree in the case described above. Cultural beliefs on both sides can also lead to misunderstandings. For example, the fear and guilt that masturbation may have been 'weakening' seems particularly strong in some Asian men. There may also be different expectations about the woman's role and about arranged marriages. It becomes even more important than usual for the doctor to listen with an open mind to what the patient says and feels.

BEING 'GOOD ENOUGH'

Many men talk about their feeling of inadequacy in their failure to control their ejaculation, expressing their fear of the woman's anger even though she may not be complaining. If such men can leave the consulting room with the sense that the doctor finds them good enough, they may be able to feel good enough at home, reducing anxiety and increasing their confidence enough to improve their symptom.

A 37-year-old man telephoned for an appointment and said, 'It's about premature ejaculation. Do you remember my wife and I came before about pregnancy?' Their GP had referred them because the wife had been ambivalent about giving up her career, while he very much wanted to become a father. At the first appointment they seemed confident in their eventual decision to try for a pregnancy. They both enjoyed sex, and so thought they would enjoy trying. Six months later the wife had not conceived and they were referred for investigation of infertility. The couple became disappointed and gave up trying. Another year passed and they considered adoption, but finally decided to throw themselves into their careers instead.

When the doctor asked the man if he might have some resentful feelings about his wife because she did not want to persevere, he replied, 'Oh no! The fault was with me. I had very few sperm, although the count did improve after some injections.' On thinking carefully about when the loss of ejaculation control started, he said, 'It was when Elizabeth stopped wanting to reach orgasm. Now she doesn't bother about it, whereas before she really enjoyed it. I failed her over this pregnancy, and now I don't even give her an orgasm.' The doctor pointed out that it was Elizabeth who had withdrawn in the relationship and not he — that a vicious circle was created and he was blaming himself. 'You seem to take the blame for everything.' He agreed that he did, and began to reflect that perhaps she was entitled to change her needs, which was not necessarily an attack on him, so he need not feel guilty.

In the interview it was clear that this couple's grief over their childlessness was unhealed. This was discussed with the man by the doctor, who was able to share the fact of the inappropriate way of dealing with his resentments.

BEHAVIOURAL OR INTERPRETIVE THERAPY?

Many books on sex therapy describe the 'squeeze technique' for training in control of ejaculation, but couples abound who have tried it and are still in trouble. The woman is instructed to caress the penis while her partner lies on his back. He concentrates on the feelings produced, and tells her when ejaculation is imminent. She then grasps the penis, encircling it with fingers and thumb at the junction of the glans with the shaft, and presses firmly. The erection should then fade. This is repeated several times and the man tries to gain control, but many say that ejaculation comes anyway.

In psychological terms, the squeeze technique can be seen as a powerful woman teaching an immature man how to switch his sexual drive on and off. When it works, as has been reported by Masters and Johnson (1970) and others, the man manages to abdicate his wishes to be in charge of the woman for the time being, and get them back later.

Men who do not respond to a woman masturbating them are unconsciously inhibiting arousal, disappointing the woman as they may have rebelliously disappointed their mother during their early life. Other reasons for failure include the partner sabotaging the man's efforts by antagonism or disinterest.

In order for behavioural techniques to be successful it is essential that the doctor sees both members of the couple. In some centres, two therapists are used so each partner can have his or her 'own' therapist. It seems likely that the success of the method depends on subtle changes in the unconscious interpersonal power balance between the couple that was mentioned at the beginning of this chapter.

When brief interpretive therapy with the man only is successful, he will begin to react differently in the relationship at home (p. 32). It is then not usually necessary for the doctor to see the partner.

Many men manage to get round their problem without understanding it by making love a second time an hour or so later if they are able to. They report less prematurity. Some masturbate before intercourse and are less excitable the second time.

NON-EJACULATION

The problem of non-ejaculation includes those men who have never ejaculated, even in their sleep, as well as those who can have wet dreams but who cannot ejaculate when they masturbate. Others can masturbate when they are alone, but cannot do so in the presence of a woman, nor respond to her touching. Others can ejaculate normally except within the vagina. The problem of non-ejaculation is more common than is generally realized.

Men often keep this difficulty to themselves for a long time, but eventually some seek help in order to obtain sexual pleasure. Others only seek help in response to their partner's dissatisfaction, or because of their wish for a pregnancy. These men are motivated for change only because of the needs of their partner. They may have consulted their GP, the family planning clinic, the clinic for urogenital disease, the gynaecologist's out-patients, or the specialist psychosexual clinic. Once again, the symptom may be primary or secondary, and while originating in the unconscious, can sometimes be helped by a brief psychosexual approach.

A 17-year-old student asked his GP for help with a failure of ejaculation on masturbation. He was referred to a urologist, who wrote that the symptom was probably psychosomatic because although the boy thought he needed circumcision because of a tight foreskin, on examination everything was normal. This intelligent, fair-haired schoolboy talked about sticking with boys at parties, and the fear of being left alone with a girl. 'If I ever get close to one, she'll know that I can't ejaculate, and what a fool I will feel then.'

During three interviews the doctor learned about Philip's divorced parents and the pressure he felt to be the man of the house for his mother and older sister. He had talked about his problem with his father, who had advised him to see his GP. He had been keen for his male GP to examine his penis, but it was only at the third psychosexual interview that the female doctor realized that an examination had not been suggested. Philip had an air of immaturity and ignorance about sexual matters, and when the doctor suggested he should get on the couch, he looked very anxious. 'You're not keen for me to look?' she asked. 'I might be dirty,' he said, revealing a fear that the doctor might find his body unattractive. The doctor noticed that when asked to push the foreskin back he handled the penis as if it were very fragile. He agreed that in fact, it was not tight, but remarked that a friend had told him that when he first had intercourse it would hurt, and would also be painful for the girl. The verbalization of this fear enabled the doctor to say, 'It seems as though you have great anxiety about vaginas too.' To which he replied, 'I don't know anything about them.'

It was tempting for the doctor to become the educator. Whereas most boys of 17 would be able to find out such things for themselves, his was a special kind of ignorance, perhaps from having been expected to 'know', as the man of the house. Philip soon failed to keep an appointment, but sent a letter saying, 'On Monday I had an orgasm while masturbating for the first time and have managed to repeat it with remarkable ease. It's true that I didn't want to before and I'm not sure that I'm happy now that I have.'

In this doctor/patient relationship the boy was able to discuss his uncertainties about sexuality. His specific fears of pain and of causing pain were revealed during the genital examination. He was then able to begin to release his sexual feelings when he was by himself, and hopefully would be able to continue the growing up process. The doctor was given no further opportunity to explore his remaining uncertainties, and, as is so often the case with psychosexual work, had to accept that she would not know the end results of her intervention.

A detailed study of 22 men (Lincoln and Thexton, 1983) who were unable to ejaculate found that even those who improved gave their female doctors a difficult time, not being able to give them any credit for the improvement. Those who did not improve tended to raise expectations of success in the doctor, only to frustrate her at the end.

SELF-MOTIVATION

A 30-year-old man was brought to the clinic by his girl-friend, who spoke for him while he looked very embarrassed. 'I live with him and we love each other very much, but when we have sex he doesn't "come"; he says he nearly does.' The doctor looked at Martin and said, 'You let her speak for you?' 'It *is* my problem,' he said. The girl went back into the waiting room, and Martin then poured out a lot about himself, almost like an ejaculation, the facts following each other in a rush. 'I used to think that I'd end up as a bachelor; I never knew any girls until I met Julia, who works in my father's business. We get on very well and she sleeps with me in my flat over the shop, which I manage for my father. The trouble is that my father has a key and sometimes he comes in at any time to discuss business, and he looks shocked if he sees Julia there.' He went on to say that he was bullied at his big comprehensive school, and so truanted and did not get any O levels, but that it did not matter as he was good at the business, in fact better than his father. 'He's getting past it and he relies on me because he's forgetful.' He said that Julia took the Pill, but that he was too shy to ask her if she took it regularly, and worried terribly that she would get pregnant. Later she assured him that she was protected. After a long pause Martin said, 'I think it's because I've masturbated from early on in an unusual way – by squeezing the root of my penis between my legs. I think this has damaged me. I've never told anybody about this before.' The doctor felt this was the moment for a genital examination, and Martin appeared very pleased when he was told there was no physical damage. Julia came back into the room and looked surprised that Martin appeared relieved and comfortable. The doctor felt a great block had been pushed aside, and Martin would be able to ejaculate from now on.

At the next visit, a month later, however, Martin was no better. He had put a lock on the flat door to keep his father out, but still felt uncomfortable when his father showed displeasure at Julia staying in the flat. He could not lead a free sexual life without his father's approval. It embarrassed him when his friends kept asking him for the date of his wedding. 'I need to be quite sure, and Julia doesn't want to settle down anyway.' At the third visit he expressed many critical feelings about Julia – her untidiness, her habit of leaving the washing-up, and the food uncovered. He used to enjoy jogging on his own, but Julia does not like him to go and so he has given it up. He described some of Julia's friends as 'drop-outs'. He himself had always worked hard and could not live in a squat as they did. He felt that his elder brother was his parents' favourite, being clever and musical. 'In the middle of sex my mind wanders off and thinks of mundane things. Sex was awful yesterday; in the middle I remembered that I had to come to the clinic and it put me off.' The doctor's early optimism faded, and the next appointment was deferred for two months so Martin would not feel pressured to make progress; he seemed to be rejecting the possibility of change.

Martin is an example of those patients who only seek help because their partner demands it. The woman is cheated of pleasure in his orgasm and of the possibility of conceiving, and although the man can maintain an erection in long and active intercourse, the partner may say, 'He goes on and on and seems not to be making love to me, but performs it as a chore.' In the doctor/patient relationship the unconscious hostility and inhibition of honest aggression can be recognized by the way in which the man makes the doctor feel optimistic and then disappointed – just as he does in intercourse with the woman.

Fear of commitment can cause inhibition of ejaculation in some men. In Martin's case, for example, it seemed he was most keen to talk about his father, and his feelings towards Julia were very ambivalent.

Secondary non-ejaculation may follow divorce or the death of a wife. If the grieving process has not been worked through there may be unconscious feelings of disloyalty towards the deceased. One man who had looked after his children for three years after his wife's death felt he would find it very difficult to share the parenting role. Ejaculation was all right with casual friends, but when he met a woman who was important to him he ran into difficulties he could not overcome, until he was able to get in touch with his anxieties about her future relationship with his children.

RELUCTANT FATHERS

Some men have a distaste for fatherhood that is openly expressed, but others find plausible reasons such as the mortgage or job, or a planned holiday to explain why it is 'inconvenient just now'. Some men will cease to ejaculate if their partner stops taking the Pill in order to become pregnant, or they may not be able to ejaculate at the fertile time of her cycle. Men who have had a bad experience of their wife's childbirth may be inhibited by it. One Jamaican man described vividly being with his mother during childbirth and seeing the blood and pain. He had sought help because he could not ejaculate when he and his girlfriend wished for a baby. Sharing his memories of his mother's pain helped him to put it behind him, and the problem had a happy outcome.

Men who have difficulty in taking on the role of fathers may have had an unsatisfactory father model with which to identify. The father may have been an alcoholic, absent from home, or not sufficiently potent in the marriage to help the boy to progress from being his mother's son, with the need to adapt to her wishes, to the role of an independent man and fatherhood. Men who feel uncertain about their own value may see a baby as a rival for their wife's attention, and unconsciously do not wish to come second. In the study mentioned earlier (Lincoln and Thexton, 1983) seven of the 22 men had been born a twin (13 times the national incidence), and many others talked about siblings of whom they had been very jealous.

In successful intercourse each partner shares closely with the other. The man gains from the woman a warm, exciting, giving vagina, and she from the man the pleasure of his penis within her. Each is aroused and responsive. The man does not give the woman an orgasm; they both have to feel safe enough in the vulnerability of letting their feelings show. Ejaculatory difficulties occur when there are unconscious feelings about women, which cause anxiety or hostility towards them. Boys learn to relate to women through interaction with the important women in their early lives. When his mother's dominance continues into adulthood, a man is held back from experiencing his sexuality in a rewarding way. He may spill his semen too soon, or he may withhold it, frustrating his partner and often being destructive of his own joy of sharing.

The doctor's role is to help these men to understand their

48 *Ejaculatory difficulties*

unconscious needs so they can relinquish them. The work may be difficult and unrewarding, and the woman doctor in particular should not expect thanks. Those men who are able to reward a woman do not appear for therapy, for in their own setting they are already making their woman 'happy enough'. The reward is a patient who no longer needs the doctor because he has been able to sort out his problem.

REFERENCES

Bancroft, J. (1989) *Human Sexuality and its Problems*, 2nd edn, Churchill Livingston, Edinburgh.
Kinsey, A. C., Pomeroy, W. B. and Martin, C. E. (1948) *Sexual Behaviour in the Human Male*, W. R. Saunders, Philadelphia.
Lincoln, R. and Thexton, R. (1983) Retarded ejaculation, in *Practice of Psychosexual Medicine* (Ed. K. Draper), J. Libbey, London.
Masters, W. H. and Johnson, V. E. (1970) *Human Sexual Inadequacy*, J & A Churchill Ltd, London.

5

The management of perversions, with special reference to transvestitism

Mervin Glasser

SUMMARY

- Transvestitism
- Differential diagnosis
- The core complex
- Treatment and management

Patients suffering from perversions present in a wide variety of ways. While they may complain of their perversions explicitly and ask for something to be done to be rid of them, more commonly the complaint is of the consequences of these conditions. Such patients may present complaining of psychosexual dysfunction, insomnia, or depression; or they may present with physical symptoms, either as the result of masochistic sexual practices, or as psychosomatic complaints which may be the consequences of such conditions.

Because these conditions are identified by the nature of the sexual act involved – 'homosexual', 'transvestite', 'child abuser'

This chapter is an extended version of a paper given at the autumn meeting of the Institute of Psychosexual Medicine on 2 November 1990.

and so on – a false impression of homogeneity is conveyed. It should be kept in mind that there are different kinds of homosexual (Limentani, 1977), child abuser (Glasser, 1979a), and so on. At the same time, our study of these conditions has led us to recognize that irrespective of their outward form, they belong to a specific diagnostic group, like 'psychoses', 'neuroses', and others, defined by a common psychodynamic structure. For want of a better, less pejorative, term we continue to refer to them as 'the perversions', as distinct from 'sexual deviations'. The latter is essentially a statistical term, which on the basis of frequency establishes a norm, any difference from which is a deviation. In this sense we are all sexually deviant since we all have our personal, idiosyncratic sexual styles and preferences. Sexual deviations may or may not be secondary to other conditions, such as psychoses, whereas perversions are a specific, primary diagnostic category.

An understanding of the common psychodynamic structure of the perversions is essential: on such an understanding depends reliable diagnostic assessment and the treatment and management based on this. The treatment of the perversions is fraught with difficulties, and should only be carried out by adequately trained persons; however, this does not preclude primary care from providing invaluable aid and relief.

TRANSVESTITISM

Main features
The general remarks above may be illustrated through a consideration of transvestitism, or cross-dressing.

Cross-dressing is as old as man himself – or at least as old as sexually differentiated clothing. Herodotus (b. 484 BC) referred to this condition as the 'Skythian illness', so named after the Skythians, a people who lived on the Black Sea. When affected, hitherto 'normal' men would put on female clothes, do women's work and generally behave in a feminine way. In commenting on this behaviour, Hippocrates assumed it was due to the mechanical trauma to these men's genitalia incurred by excessive horse riding, for which they were well known. Achilles cross-dressed, although this was for concealment in the court of Lycomedes, to which he was sent by his mother to prevent him from going to the Trojan War, where she knew he would perish (Wright, 1978).

Cross-dressing may fall within normal boundaries, such as the dressing-up for fancy dress parties and that commonly carried out by young children. Such cross-dressing needs to be differentiated from transvestitism, which is a perversion.

> A typical example of a transvestite was Mr W, a 29-year-old man seen at the Portman Clinic, and subsequently in full analysis privately. His transvestite act consisted of dressing up as a woman, paying careful attention to the minutest details – the exact size and shape of the padding put into his brassière and the precise tightness of its straps; the smoothness of the texture of the panties and the feel of their tightness round his waist; the matching blouse and skirt, tights, and shoes; the hairstyle of the wig; and so on – all to ensure that what he saw in the mirror was a neatly and attractively dressed woman. It was important there was nothing in his appearance and bodily feel to dispel this experience of himself as a woman. For example, he could not wear his ordinary wristwatch, even if this was hidden by the sleeve of his blouse. Mr W would then masturbate looking at himself in the mirror, arranging himself in such a way that his penis was not visible in the reflection. (Glasser, 1979a).

Apart from the sexual pleasure Mr W derived from this activity, it also gave him a feeling of relaxation and a sense of freedom, and it relieved him of any aggressive feelings. Mr W belonged to the group of transvestites who are extremely concerned to keep their activities secret, in contrast to others who have a strong desire to appear in female garb in public (see also Stoller, 1974).

DIFFERENTIAL DIAGNOSIS

The transvestite thus cross-dresses as his preferred, if not exclusive, way of obtaining sexual gratification. This needs to be differentiated from other cross-dressing activities reflecting abnormality. In contrast to the transvestite, the transsexual derives no sexual arousal or pleasure from cross-dressing, but regards it simply as wearing the appropriate clothing for his 'true' gender identity. Whereas the transvestite suffers from the castration anxiety that all men experience (Freud, 1926), the transsexual does not – in fact he energetically seeks castration (Limentani, 1979; Stoller, 1975). The fetishist is typically aroused by women's clothing, but this is generally limited to one specific item, such as high-heeled shoes, underwear, and so on, and he generally prefers the article/s to be worn by his sexual partner rather than by himself. The homosexual may dress up in women's clothes, but this is not in itself sexually exciting; it may, however, arouse sexual interest in other homosexuals. While the transvestite idealizes the woman he is trying to look and feel like, there is an element of mockery of women in the homosexual's dressing up. Perhaps it needs emphasizing that the transvestite does not entertain any homosexual desires, and in fact energetically resists any suggestion that this element may be part of his make-up.

Table 5.1 *Differentiating features of different forms of cross-dressing*

Feature	Transvestite	Transsexual	Fetishist	Homosexual
Clothing	Must be female	Must be female	Predominantly female	Occasionally female
Specificity of clothing	Not limited	Not limited	Limited to specific item	Not limited
Where worn	On own body	On own body	Usually on other's body	On own body
Love object	Female	Male, if at all	Female	Male
Sexual excitement	Yes	No	Yes	No
Castration anxiety	Yes	No	Yes	Yes
Transsexual wish	Variable, but No ultimately	Yes	No	No

It may be noted that apart from homosexuality and transsex-ualism, which is not a perversion, these conditions are to all intents and purposes not found in females. Though women may wear articles of men's clothing, this does not occur as the preferred or exclusive form of sexual arousal and fulfilment.

No reliable figures of incidence can be given because cross-dressing is often carried out secretly, and it is not known how many transvestites never seek medical or other help. Table 5.2 gives the numbers of patients suffering from perversions seen at the Portman Clinic in the period 1976–78. Though this may be regarded as reflecting the incidence in the general population, this can only be in the crudest way since there are so many factors which determine a referral to the Clinic.

Table 5.2 *Incidence of perversions seen at the Portman Clinic 1976–78 (Glasser, 1990)*

Perversion	Number of patients seen ($n=746$)
Transvestites	47 (6%)
Fetishists	44 (6%)
Homosexuals	257 (35%)
Paedophiles	102 (14%)
Other	296 (40%)

Family background

The typical family background of the transvestite is one in which the mother played a dominant role. Though she was a conscientious mother who provided good material care for the child, she was involved emotionally only insofar as her son served her psychological needs; that is, she related to him narcissistically. It is almost pathognomonic of the transvestite that his mother wanted a daughter, and it is not unusual for the patient to report that as a child he was dressed in girl's clothes and had his hair done in a girl's style. The father is a rather shadowy figure in the patient's accounts, and features as emotionally distant, even absent.

THE CORE COMPLEX

The psychodynamic structure of the perversions is extremely complicated, receiving as it does contributions from all parts of the personality. It is useful to conceptualize this structure by visualizing a model of a large, elaborate molecule made up of numerous component complexes, each complex containing elements interacting with each other, and each complex relating dynamically to the others. At the heart of this molecule is a component complex that exercises a predominant and pervasive influence on all the other component complexes. I have termed it the 'Core Complex' (Glasser, 1979a). Because of considerations of space, I shall limit this discussion to the significance of this complex in the psychopathology of perversions.

Two types of violence
Before elaborating the constituent elements of the core complex, it is useful to consider some aspects of violence, since these play a crucial role in the nature of perversions.

Violence is something fundamental, something built into us by biology – it is the active expression of the body's basic reaction pattern which prepares it for 'fight-or-flight' in the presence of danger (Cannon, 1953). The danger that provokes this integrated response is anything that is a threat to survival; the aim of the violent act is to destroy or negate the danger. In humans, this 'self-preservative' violence is provoked far more frequently by threats to a person's psychological status and integrity than by physical dangers. Each of us has a sense of 'Self': a separate, independent identity whose integrity and worth we protect with as much vehemence as we do our physical existence. Any threat to the self will automatically provoke self-preservative violence unless there are modifying or inhibiting influences. This violence aims at negating the danger to the self, just as when the danger is physical.

In addition to self-preservative violence we may distinguish a second major category of violence: malicious or sadistic violence. This has as its aim the infliction of physical and emotional suffering. There is no aim to destroy the object of the violence. The most clear-cut example of malicious violence is sexual sadism. We are all familiar with examples of violence where, although explicit sexual excitement is not evident, the pleasure in cruelly inflicting pain is quite obvious.

The perpetrator's attitude to the victim is the most immediate way of distinguishing these two forms of violence: in self-preservative violence the aim is to negate the danger; apart from this, the victim's experience of the act, his emotional reaction, his fate in any other respect, is irrelevant. In sadistic violence, on the other hand, the emotional reaction of the victim is crucial: the specific aim is to cause suffering, physically or mentally, crudely or subtley.

The desire for fusion and the fear of annihilation
To return now to the core complex. What we are able to observe in the psychotherapy of individuals suffering from perversions is a usually unacknowledged but deeply felt longing to form a permanent union of profound intimacy with another person, amounting to a fusion with that person. This fusion fantasy contains a wish for complete satisfaction of all needs, and for absolute security against any danger of deprivation or attack. It also has a containing quality, guarding against feelings of disintegration, or loss of control of violent or other impulses. This desire for an all-giving, all-embracing person points to the persistence into adulthood of attitudes and expectations of early development: the core complex initially is experienced by the infant in relation to its mother.

Such desires for fusion are by no means foreign to the most normal of people. But what distinguishes the type of person being considered is that for him or her such a union does not have the character of a temporary state; he is deeply convinced, more unconsciously than consciously, that it would be a permanent fusion, involving an irrevocable and irreversible loss of self. What for a normal person would be a deeply satisfying but transient union, with an enrichment of his/her own sense of worth and identity, is for such a disturbed person a disappearance of his separate, independent existence into that of the other person.

There are innumerable variations in how such individuals conceive of this loss of self: one will regard coming close to the other person as resulting in engulfment or envelopment by that person; another will conceive of it as being 'intruded into' or possessed; another as a passive merging; and so on. Physical and emotional closeness are, in one way or another, perceived as inevitably leading to being taken over totally by the other person; the fulfilment of his intense longings for fusion must ultimately involve a total annihilation of his self. As one patient expressed this, it is 'like sugar dissolving in a cup of coffee'.

Withdrawal and the fear of abandonment
What the pervert believes to be the intrinsic consequence of closeness leads him to respond with the basic flight-or-fight reaction. The flight reaction consists of withdrawal, essentially into himself. However, this brings isolation and deprivation from the very emotional supplies for which he so intensely longs. In addition, because of the resultant loss of the containing capacities of the longed-for person, fear of loss of control and bodily disintegration may also be experienced. The individual will consequently suffer strong feelings of depression, insignificance, worthlessness, and desolation. Feeling alienated and abandoned, he experiences an intensifying desire to return to the object of his longings, which culminate in wishes for a complete and reassuringly indissoluble union, which is the starting point of this part of the core complex. This part of the core complex, therefore, can be seen to have the nature of a vicious circle.

Self-preservative violence and the fear of loss
Coming close to the longed-for union, with its increasingly intense threat of annihilation, provokes both withdrawal and an increasingly intense propulsion to self-preservative violence, as well as intense anxiety – the fight component of the fight-or-flight response. At its extreme this would be aimed at destroying the dangerous, albeit longed-for, other person. However, this other person (originally the mother) is at the same time the focus of the individual's deepest longings and emotional needs.

These then are the most prominent features of the core complex: the longing for complete fusion, with the consequent development of annihilation anxiety and impulses to self-preservative violence. There is also withdrawal, with consequent feelings of abandonment, anxiety, agitated depression, low self-esteem, and fears of disintegration. The core complex is thus characterized by intense and conflicting motives and reactions.

Resolution of the conflicts
How the pervert solves this dilemma is a key step in the formation of the perversion: through a process of sexualization, the negating, self-preservative violence is converted into malicious or sadistic violence. The result of this is the preservation of the other person

(originally the mother) who is no longer threatened by total destruction because the intention to destroy is converted into the wish to hurt and control. Since this also involves an exclusion of the drive towards merging with the other person the danger of annihilation no longer threatens. The viability of the relationship thus is ensured, albeit henceforth always on a sado-masochistic footing. This is why sado-masochism is an essential and invariable characteristic of the pervert's relationships. And when we study other component complexes of the perversions, we see how they are affected – we might say distorted – by this outcome of the core complex.

The features of the core complex may be discerned in the perverse act. For example, in the case of Mr W, cross-dressing is carried out with the aim of experiencing himself to be a woman, that is, of giving gratification in concrete, bodily terms of being fused with the woman, originally his mother. Mr W felt that by experiencing what a woman experiences through her body, he could persuade himself he had become her. At the same time, his act of masturbation emphatically reassures him of his masculinity and the presence of his penis, as a counter to castration anxiety.

However, since Mr W's act of imagined bodily fusion raises annihilation anxiety, he needs to feel the freedom to escape, whenever he so wishes, something he can do in the context of his perverse act by undressing. Thus undressing is as important a component of the perverse act as dressing. The cross-dressing is also experienced as keeping in check any violence he may be feeling, by carrying out the process of sexualizing the self-preservative violence. For example, when Mr W became furious with a friend of his and felt he wanted to assault him savagely, he rushed off to the wash-basket in the bathroom and put on some of his wife's clothing, rapidly becoming calm and relaxed.

It will be seen that ultimately the pervert's solution is unsuccessful: he is unable to establish and maintain genuinely intimate and lasting relationships; the other person always threatens to be experienced as an annihilator; the distressing reactions such as murderous rage, depression, poor self-esteem, and instability are always present or potentially present. It is this unresolved outcome of the core complex conflicts, as well as others arising from other parts of the whole structure, which leads to the assertion that the perversions are morbid conditions, and not just a less common way of achieving love and sexual gratification.

TREATMENT AND MANAGEMENT

By focusing on the core complex and the aetiological factors associated with it, it is possible to gain an impression of the dynamic interplay of powerful psychological needs. It can therefore be appreciated that while psychotherapy of such patients is too substantial an undertaking except for the experienced psychotherapist in the field, competent management may be carried out with confidence if the underlying psychodynamic situation is kept in mind.

Perhaps of most importance for immediate practical application is the recognition that the pervert is driven by most primal and painful emotional needs, rather than by simple sexual desire. It helps us to develop a perspective on the compulsive 'cottaging' (going into public toilets to make brief, promiscuous sexual contacts) of some homosexuals, the desperate stealing from clothes-lines of some transvestites and fetishists, the evident incorrigibility of the indecent exposers. We see that so often their sexual behaviour, sometimes described as addictive in nature, is driven by a search for the relief of psychic pain rather than by a desire for pleasure, although the special nature of sexual pleasure is indisputably an essential ingredient.

The doctor's role

A maintenance contact with the patient – seeing him from time to time rather than on a more frequent, intensive basis – may be very helpful and effective. Bearing in mind the annihilation anxieties, the doctor needs to keep a more careful check on himself in his dealings with the pervert patient than he would need to do with others. Maintaining a professional distance, without taking it to the extreme where it could be experienced as hostile, would actually be reassuring to the pervert, even though he may grumble about the doctor's aloofness or remoteness. At the same time, the giving of clear and reliable appointments may give the patient a sense of stability and security, which could counteract the development of any abandonment anxieties. The underlying principle is that of the great value of the maintenance contact in providing a firm, reliable, but unconfining structure.

Another consideration derives from the pervert's special relationship to his superego which is experienced as an inner person rather than as abstract concepts and feelings of right and wrong, good and bad, ideal or contemptible. This inner person is related to in the same core complex terms as people in the external world. Thus, he is governed by the belief that achieving a harmony with his conscience, fulfilling his ideals, being 'good' are regarded as submitting to, and thus being taken over by, the superego – again with an inevitable, as he believes, annihilation of the self. The demands of the superego are thus openly or covertly defied.

Because the doctor features as such an authority figure the pervert-patient *must* at some point defy the doctor's efforts, however selfless they might be. Here we see a second reason for such patients' tendencies not to co-operate with their helpers. The patient may miss appointments or come late, or he may become distracted just when the doctor is saying something of particular importance; in innumerable ways he defies or evades what he regards as the doctor's instructions or demands. This may present insuperable impediments to constructive work with such patients.

The doctor, however, can do much to minimize or even avoid such difficulties. He needs to be careful not to pressure the patient into following some course of action, however valuable the doctor may judge it to be. The doctor should avoid passing judgemental comments, positive or negative. He needs to try to counter, or at least not to confirm, being cast in the role of the superego in the transference by examining his own motivation, differentiating between his true role as a doctor, rather than his perhaps idealistic role as an improver of society. So necessary and deeply established are the dynamics of the pervert's make-up that it would be unrealistic to expect him to change substantially simply on the basis of his being in distress or on the basis of wise advice offered to him by his doctor.

A feature of the pervert-patient that can place great strain on the doctor is his characteristic sado-masochistic way of object-relating, which is brought into the relationship with the doctor. In obvious or subtle ways he can seek to make the doctor look ridiculous or incompetent; or he can attempt to cast himself in the role of the failure or in a helpless and hopeless situation. At times he may contrive to be the victim of the doctor's mismanagement, for example, making a suicide attempt following the doctor's refusal to prescribe inappropriate medication. Here again steadfastness of structure and awareness of the limited aims of the contact can prove to be much more helpful than might initially be anticipated in dealing with the sado-masochistic manoeuvres.

Perhaps the most difficult issue for the doctor to cope with is when something in the patient's material is sexually arousing, when it touches on a perhaps not readily acknowledged aspect of the doctor's own psychosexual make-up. It need not be said that it is not therapeutically beneficial for such an issue either to be pursued or censored: if there is any feeling of insecurity in the management of this, it is best to refer the patient to another professional.

The enduring value of primary care

There are a number of different therapeutic approaches to the perversions. Only the Portman Clinic in Great Britain and, as far as I know, in the world specifically caters for such patients, offering psychoanalytic psychotherapy. But the perversions are a particularly difficult group to treat, and therapy of any nature is not always successful. The role of the primary carer will thus always be a vital one. Given an adequate conception of the psychodynamic ingredients of such a patient's make-up, primary care can make a particularly valuable contribution.

REFERENCES

Cannon, W. B. (1953) *Bodily Changes in Pain, Hunger, Fear and Rage*, Charles T. Branford Company, Boston.

Freud, S. (1926) Inhibitions, symptoms and anxiety, in the Standard Edition of the *Complete Psychological Works of Sigmund Freud*, vol. 20, Hogarth Press, London, pp. 72–175.

Glasser, M. (1979a) From the analysis of a transvestite. *Int. Rev. Psycho-Anal.*, 6, 163–73.

Glasser, M. (1979b) Some aspects of the role of aggression in the perversions, in *Sexual Deviation*, 2nd edn (Ed. I. Rosen), Oxford University Press, Oxford, pp. 278–305.

Glasser, M. (1990) Paedophilia, in *Principles and Practice of Forensic Psychiatry* (Ed. R. Bluglass and P. Bowden), Churchill Livingstone, London, pp. 739–48.

Limentani, A. (1979) The significance of transsexualism in relation to some basic psychoanalytic concepts. *Int. Rev. Psycho-Anal.*, 6, 139–53.

Stoller, R. (1974) *Sex and Gender*, Jacob Aronson, New York.

Stoller, R. (1975) *The Transsexual Experiment*, Hogarth Press, London.

Wright, F. A. (1978) *Lemprière's Classical Dictionary of Proper Names* mentioned in *Ancient Authors*, Routledge & Kegan Paul, London.

6

Male sexual development: a psychological view

Gill Hinshelwood

SUMMARY

- The earliest days
- Infantile sexuality
- Envy
- The father's influence
- Rivalry with father
- Developmental influences on adult sexuality

A man who had been treated for impotence told the doctor on his last visit that he had actually registered under a false name because he had been so embarrassed about his difficulty. The name he had chosen for himself was Mr Mann. The doctor commented that he had clearly expressed both his problem and his hopes in choosing the name. The patient said in amazement, 'But I just plucked it out of thin air; it was the first name that came to mind'. The status of manhood is related very closely to sexual performance, and this impotent patient felt he had lost his manhood. It is important to stress, however, that his manhood felt lost in relation to women.

How does the baby boy develop into a sexual adult male, and what are the vicissitudes he encounters on the way?

THE EARLIEST DAYS

Under normal circumstances, on birth the infant is received into the arms of a warm and loving mother. The helpless and immature baby is entirely dependent on this all-important person to meet his every need. Everything he takes in comes from her, and everything he evacuates goes to her. The first object he sees is her face leaning over him, and the first object he touches is her breast. When she smiles, he smiles, and when she coos he coos, and the mother responds to the infant's reciprocation.

This blissful dyad could go on forever, and with it such mutual identification that mother and baby would grow more and more in the image of the other. A state of mind can exist in which mother and baby each feel themselves to be an extension of the other. At moments of bliss this is a deeply rewarding and enriching experience, but there is a dreadful corollary for the baby, for whom there are two objects: the infinitely loving, containing, mother who is present, but also a painful, hateful mother who is absent. This is a very frightening time for the baby, when the complete world in which he thought he was king, able to conjure up milk and warmth from a source within his power, has disappeared, and with it himself.

Fortunately, things change rapidly and as the baby grows, nurtured by mother, his field of vision widens and mother becomes more real. She is no longer just an experience, but another person who is sometimes there, making life safe and contented, but also a person who is sometimes not there, bringing pain and despair. In this way the beginning of self and other are experienced, with all its terrifying implications, as well as the beginning of love and hate.

As the weeks go by, these two key figures – present mother and absent mother – slowly merge and mother becomes one and the same person. The baby realizes he is adoring the same warm and nurturing woman that he is also hating. With this realization the child is confronted with a profound dilemma: can mother survive his violent attacks, his greed, his destruction, and will she ever come back? Has his anger gone too far, and will his love and gratitude be enough to make amends? The child experiences all this without the words to ask, and without the comprehension of words for the answer.

The baby who thought he was in charge, that milk flowed at his command realizes he is only a helpless little baby, completely dependent on the whims of a fickle woman. This can have frightening implications. The symbiotic state of the early weeks can be experienced by the baby as existing only when his mother is there, leaving a terrifying feeling of 'not being' when she is absent. There can be despair that he is really nothing and no one, and he can feel anger and wounded pride. However, in his ability to be welcoming and pleased when he is picked up, and to smile and give something back, he realizes his distressed and angry outbursts have not killed off his mother; she still comes back. Gradually the anguish of this period for the baby is lessened, the depression and guilt become bearable, and the next developmental task begins.

INFANTILE SEXUALITY

How does sexuality develop? A baby boy or girl is a bundle of sensual feeling, and every event such as sucking, making eye contact, being picked up and handled, being kissed, is pleasurable. A baby lying replete and satisfied, in touch with his mother's breast, is in ecstasy, and mirrored in the mother's face is that same satisfaction.

The earliest organs of sensory pleasure are the mouth and lips, with which the baby derives the satisfaction of sucking the nipple, taking in food, and feeling objects. Evacuation of faeces is the next activity of interest, and the anus becomes the sensually dominant area of the body. The battles with mother are over the triumphant pleasures of giving and withholding, control and domination, and of closeness and separateness. These are real battles; the toddler shows an active interest in mess and has no shame, wishing for sadistic pleasure and controlling omnipotence in relation to mother, the first woman in his life.

The developing boy's discovery of his penis as a potent source of pleasure is the most satisfying discovery of all: it is a secret comfort that is available when he is alone and unstimulated, whereas the other pleasures are dependent on another person. In the self-creation of states of pleasure the baby adds his own fantasies gleaned from his interaction with the world, or with his mother, who constitutes his whole world during the earliest months.

Although these are the earliest days in the life of a man or a woman, already the infant has felt the intensities of loving and of murderous passion; of terror and despair, which may be revived many times in later years, and even equalled, but never surpassed.

ENVY

The little boy loves and admires this wonderful mother who does everything for him, but he may also feel very envious of her creativity, of her abundant milk, which he at first thought he made himself. Even the wonderful ability of the mother to love and not bear grudges, as he does, can be envied rather than a welcome gift. He may hate the mother for being better at these things, and because it is dangerous the hatred may be locked away, only to emerge later in his adult relationships. He may scorn a woman's love, belittle her ability to have babies, and deny that he would like to be loved by a woman. In adulthood many men feel ambivalent about loving women. They are attracted by the love and warmth they experienced as children, repelled by the fear of female power over them, and anxious because of an unresolved fear of being abandoned.

THE FATHER'S INFLUENCE

The young infant is tolerant of other adults who are around him and who are kind to him. They play their part and are enjoyed. But after mother, the next most important adult on the scene is father – another man, like himself. At first father may be a more shadowy figure than mother – a benign person who provides for baby and mother. If father is good and attentive, the baby will reward him with smiles of welcome, and love between the two will develop.

There comes the time, however, when the toddler becomes aware that mother, who he imagined only had eyes for him, has a relationship with father that excludes him. This is the cruellest blow so far. The mother/son relationship has been going from strength to strength, and this man is perceived to have an importance in his own right, to be a rival for mother's affection and to have a relationship with her that involves sexuality and the making of babies.

The intensity of loving and hating following this realization is very great. Although there is a so-called latent period, when all these early childhood experiences are forgotten, in adult life they can be revived at a stroke, with varying success or failure depending on the outcome experienced by the toddler. This is a desperate time for him; he fears he has lost mother forever and he needs much reassurance. When she is called repeatedly to the bedroom for another goodnight kiss or a glass of water, he may be pleading to know whether she really does not love him, and what is wrong with him that he does not have the magic key to satisfy her. Is it because he is too small? Was he ridiculous and silly to have imagined he could ever satisfy a woman?

RIVALRY WITH FATHER

Father is now felt to be huge, ruthless, and frightening – a power-crazed rival who will take revenge on the young upstart for having designs on his woman. To the child there is ample reason for his fear of father's retaliation. He is aware that his mother has been loving and devoted to him, and he is in the grip of the fairly primitive, cruel retaliatory processes that he has so far used to solve his own problems. At such times he shows a fear of wolves and tigers, or engines and machinery, which are coming to destroy him.

What will be destroyed? By this time the little boy has discovered his penis, and he is aware of its strength and potency; he is proud of it and gets enormous pleasure from it. He is also aware that some children do not have one. Why? How can you lose such a valuable object? Is this what a vengeful father can do? Cut off his son's penis? Deprive him forever of his potent symbol of mastery and achievement?

Resolution of the rivalry
The little boy is also aware of his love for his father, and may at times, in identification with his mother, wish to be a partner to this man. He is pulled in many ways; something must be surrendered. The outcome is to give up believing that mother should be exclusively his, and to recognize, sadly, that father came first, and that hopefully his own turn will come. If father is kind enough,

not too insecure, rejecting or jealous at this stage, there is a tremendous growth and the little boy is permitted and encouraged to grow like father, to identify with him and to realize his own difference from mother. He can even carry on thinking she is the most wonderful woman in the world, but this cannot reach its prior intensity. His love for his father and identification with him, and his knowledge that mother loves him and admires father, enable him to begin to renounce his infantile phantasies.

The little boy has three major hurdles to overcome before he reaches school age. He has so far identified with his mother, and thinks he will be the same: he believes she, like him, has a penis, and that he is like her and will have babies. However, he has to give up some of this identification with his mother and take on identifications with his father, who is his rival – both a loved and hated man. He also has to find another way of loving his mother.

By the time the child is old enough to go to school, much of the intensity of these conflicts and passions will have subsided, leaving the child able to socialize with his peers, to learn from both men and women, and to develop with confidence. He needs both his mother's love and admiration to enable him to be pleased to be a boy and to grow away from being a mirror-image of her, and his father's encouragement and willingness to share mother's love with him.

This story of rivalry and passion, of jealousy and desire that takes place in the first four to five years of a boy's life is buried and lost to conscious memory. The grown man does not remember just as 'Mr Mann' did not remember. He was reduced to impotence in his adult life at the moment when redundancy reawakened feelings of insecurity. At a time when some sexual comfort could be felt to be very containing, this was denied to the couple.

In a way, 'Mr Mann' was unconsciously recalling what it felt like to be a child in the face of his father's superior strength. It was only with difficulty that he had recovered from the blow to his pride at that early stage in his development, and he carried within a feeling that his masculinity was vulnerable to attack. When his powerful boss made him redundant, 'Mr Mann's' feelings of smallness and impotence were reawakened. These feelings had made him feel shame and humiliation as a child when he felt his mother rejected him in favour of his father, and he was disappointed and angry with her. These feelings were later unconsciously visited upon his wife, who he also believed would only want a potent man, and who would have nothing to do with a man who could not work.

When the rivalry with the father has been resolved a latency period follows. During this time the boy grows physically, gains skills, and takes risks in becoming more independent, and copies his father in a number of ways.

The next explosive stage of emotional development is puberty, when major psychological tasks are accomplished and the family prepare for a new adult member. It is a puzzling time for the boy, when his body changes shape, hair grows on his face and genitals, and his voice alters. Sexual arousal, both as an awareness of wishes, and physical sensations in his genitals, forces the boy to face his own sexuality. He has his first seminal emission, and all those buried emotions of the toddler years are stirred up and re-experienced towards mother, father, and the outside world. The authority of the father is challenged time and time again, and the boy may try to divide the parents and have mother to himself. It is another chance to work through this conflict, and finally to leave the parents to each other and choose a relationship of his own.

DEVELOPMENTAL INFLUENCES ON ADULT SEXUALITY

All these development stages have an influence on adult sexuality. For instance, the kind of woman the man chooses and how he treats her will depend on his early years.

What situations are there in adult life that mirror the developmental blocks of infants and toddlers? 'Mr Mann', as an example of lack of sexual confidence, has already been mentioned. Some men only want someone else's woman; the seduction, the defeat of a rival is all important. Some do not marry, but carry on at home being the good and dutiful son. They dare not become men for it means renouncing mother for ever, so they stay on. They may have a fantasy of a mother needing them, of her really valuing her son more than the boring, brutish father, and appear to be just waiting for their turn to come along.

There are some men who, during childhood, were so horrified, angry, and jealous of their father's sexuality with their mother that they needed to convince themselves that no woman (mother) could really want it, and that it is a filthy, wicked, depraved thing to do to an angel. The mother, and all women thereafter, remains untouchable, and the men who do these dreadful things to her should control their base natures. The father who defiles her is aggressive and brutal, and the boy grows into a virtuous man, never daring to make love in case he destroys his woman, or his ideal of her.

A variant is the man whose sexuality is split. He cannot enjoy love-making with his partner, but seeks out prostitutes instead. For him there are good women and bad women, perhaps reflecting very early preoccupations with mother as a present good person and an absent bad person.

There are some men who fear the vagina as a wide-open cave, which will take them in and never release them again. Such a fear is related to the intensity of the early, all-embracing love. The apparent possibility of merging with the mother so that all separation and individuation is lost can be highly persecutory. For such men a deep and satisfying relationship with a woman is a terrifying prospect, as well as highly desirable. They may over and over again become deeply involved with women, and then withdraw in fear, and find a new object.

The traumatically symbiotic situation described above is likely to occur if the father has not made an appropriate impact on the development of the infant. When his role has been adequate the situation of rivalry serves the boy well, for it helps him to renounce as impossible his first love, find himself as a male in his own right, and separate from his mother. He thereafter is able to approach a woman in the secure knowledge that he can love her without merging into her.

Professionals working in the field of psychological and psycho-sexual medicine will be aware of the different disturbances in sexual relationships between men and women, and can add many other examples of pain and conflict, of lack of satisfaction in sexuality, and of physical symptoms with psychological origins, such as premature ejaculation and impotence. Linking the present complaint with childhood experiences and emotions is not always possible. What is possible and available at every consultation is a doctor/patient relationship which can be reflected upon and used. The internal relationship a man has with his mother, as laid down in those early years, will be present in his current symptoms, and will show in his relationship with his doctor. There is much truth in the old wives' tale, 'If you want to know how your future husband will treat you, watch how he treats his mother.' And one can add, with caution, his doctor.

This chapter has discussed the normal development of the internal, phantasy world of the male infant, which influences his adult sexual behaviour and self-image. There are a multitude of additional factors which may have a profound effect on his development: the child may not have been wanted or loved by his mother; the father may find him a rival; or the mother may have hated men. The possibilities are endless, and thus every individual is unique. Whatever happens in reality, the developmental stages which have been described are part of human life, in which the psychological means of negotiating all such future hurdles are structured.

7

Difficulty in achieving intercourse

Katherine Draper

SUMMARY

- Presentation
- The doctor/patient relationship in non-consummation
- The genital examination
- Couples or singles

'I bet you've never seen anyone like me before, doctor!'
A slight, girlish looking woman sat leaning forward on
the edge of her chair. The Well Woman clinic notes
revealed she was 44 years old. She whispered intensely,
'It's not nice to be called a virgin.'

This chapter describes work with those who are unable to achieve
sexual intercourse; it is not that they will not, but that they cannot.
Sometimes there is a difficulty in accepting themselves as sexual
persons; more often there is an emotional block which cannot
allow penetration and full vaginal intercourse, although the person
can enjoy arousal and sexual feeling. As a patient said recently,
'The mind says one thing and the body another.' The resulting
feelings of confusion, failure, and of being different from everyone
else are illustrated in the brief incident described above.

PRESENTATION

Articles in the press, such as 'A couple unjoined in matrimony' (Rodwell, 1987), or the publication of a personal account by a sufferer (Valins, 1988), have made it possible for some patients to make a direct complaint of non-consummation. More commonly, the feeling of being a freak and a fear of ridicule lead many to seek help with a bodily symptom, or leads to the problem being discovered by chance. There is certainly nothing in a woman's appearance that will reliably suggest this problem. While many of these women who have not consummated their sexual relationships appear shy, girlish, and immature, there are others with a flamboyant sexiness which is a mask for their inner impoverishment. This mask gradually changes to a less artificial appearance once they are able to enjoy their sexuality and have no need to pretend to be a sex-kitten. There are many different cries for help which may conceal an inability to achieve full sexual intercourse.

For two years Mrs A had attended the family planning clinic regularly, taking her pills as prescribed. A new doctor noticed that various excuses, such as menstruation and 'urgent appointments' had prevented the patient from having a smear taken. The doctor suggested she seemed to be avoiding having a pelvic examination. This observation helped her to blurt out that intercourse was impossible. Her husband was now getting impatient, and they were beginning to have rows.

A patient who was attending the psychosexual problem clinic for non-consummation asked the doctor to see her sister, Mrs B, who suffered from 'terrible PMT'. Mrs B attended with her husband, and the events of the interview suggested that some of her symptoms were a response to her husband's immature behaviour. At her next visit she expressed her sorrow at her infertility. After several discussions, the doctor realized that Mrs B had not had a smear, and suggested it should be done. She burst into tears and said they had been married for 12 years and had never been able to have intercourse. It was now possible to begin to work with her true difficulty.

Neither Mrs B nor her sister had any idea of the other's complaint, which is an example of the great secrecy which surrounds this condition.

Some couples who are unable to admit that conception is an impossibility will present at an infertility clinic. In more reticent times it was not uncommon for investigations to begin before establishing whether intercourse had occurred. Occasionally the problem only emerges when desperation leads to a suicide attempt. Because of the secretive nature of the problem, a long time may elapse between the first attempt at intercourse and a request for help, but it is interesting that the length of time to presentation does not affect the outcome of treatment (Bramley *et al.*, 1981, 1983). It is important to consider carefully why they have sought help at this particular moment, as the precipitating factor will be relevant to the understanding of their difficulty.

It is sometimes said that a psychosexual approach is not suitable for those who are not good at conceptualizing their ideas, but such people may be easier to help than those who are good with words. Some almost illiterate women can give amazingly vivid descriptions of their fantasies. True ignorance and lack of education only rarely contribute to the problem, and indeed some well-educated, professional women find it difficult to admit their problem because rationally it seems so foolish.

> Nurse C was referred to the clinic with a letter saying she could not tolerate sex. At her first visit she told the doctor she fainted every time she had to be present at a vaginal examination. After working with the doctor, she was able to reveal her fears that the vagina was a brittle, narrow tube which would fragment with a searing pain on penetration. She had passed her exams and knew how other people were made; it was only herself who was different! As soon as she was able to learn the reality of the construction of her vagina she was able to enjoy intercourse. Luckily, she attended the clinic just before her gynaecology placement; she was now able to watch vaginal examinations with impunity, as she had no fears to project on to the patient.

THE DOCTOR/PATIENT RELATIONSHIP IN NON-CONSUMMATION

Whether the presentation is overt or covert, when invited to 'Tell me about it,' the patient will often talk of a block, barrier, or wall which prevents intercourse. Sometimes this barrier is expressed non-verbally, as the patient sits silently, communicating a feeling of tension; not only is her vagina forbidden to her lover, but her thoughts cannot be shared with her doctor. In response to this barrier, the doctor may feel an irresistible urge to break through and find out what it is all about, but the doctor who is driven to ask direct questions may find the answers are not helpful. Only by allowing the consultation to develop spontaneously, by listening, observing, and then making an appropriate remark, such as, 'You seem to have difficulty in talking about this', and by allowing time for a response, can confidence and insights be gained.

About one-third of patients who cannot achieve intercourse give a history of a 'previous traumatic experience'. Half of these have suffered various acts of sexual abuse, and the rest complain of painful medical examinations. In the latter case it is unlikely that the doctors concerned had meant to be rough and bullying, but their failure was to appreciate that the feelings generated in the consultation were related to the patient's fears and anxieties. This resulted in frustration for them, which provoked irritable behaviour, which in turn exacerbated the patient's previous fears.

It was her third visit to the clinic. Miss E sat, staring belligerently at the doctor. Her boyfriend had drawn his chair close to hers, and held her hand protectively. Little progress had been made; she had refused examination at previous visits on the grounds that she did not know the doctor well enough, and that she had been kept waiting 15 minutes, and was now nervous. She looked angry and tearful as she expostulated, 'I'm too young to go through all this!' The doctor, who was aware that she was being made to feel callous and bullying, waited and then said, 'Perhaps you feel too young for sex.' There was a long pause. Miss E bridled, and then said, 'The doctor made me feel awful!' There followed an account of a visit to the GP for thrush. When asked if she slept with her boyfriend she said yes, although in fact they had only slept in a bed together; she had been too tense when intercourse was attempted. The GP had insisted on taking a smear, and the attempt was painful and unsuccessful. When she could not relax the doctor became angry and said, 'I can't be bothered with people like you. Go to the nurse!' After Miss E had unburdened herself of these angry feelings, the atmosphere changed and it became possible to start to work with her on understanding her anxieties.

This encounter demonstrates the control which is exercised, often unconsciously, as a defence against penetration, over the approaches of the doctor and the partner to mental and physical closeness. With training the doctor can acquire a detached awareness of his own feelings, which may enable him to make a remark such as, 'Your story makes me feel angry; this may be something to do with the way *you* feel.' This may free the patient to be aware of her own feelings.

Although dramatic events such as incest and traumatic examinations are often blamed in the first instance, it usually emerges that this has occurred where there is already a very inhibited attitude towards sexuality.

THE GENITAL EXAMINATION

During the examination many patients show signs of extreme anxiety, clenching the knees together and arching the back. Comforting reassurance is useless, but an enabling remark such as, 'This makes you very frightened,' may help them to share the reason for their fears. To proceed and cause pain will only reinforce the idea that anything entering the vagina is painful, and so the examination must only take place at a pace that can be tolerated without too much distress. Sometimes control is an important issue, and the patient, if asked, will herself introduce the doctor's passive finger. However, it is important that the meaning of this is understood. To carry out an examination under anaesthesia will only reinforce the patient's fears, implying that the genital area can only be approached when the patient is unconscious.

Vaginismus is the name given to the spasm of the involuntary muscles of the lower third of the vagina in response to any attempted penetration. It is experienced as pain, which can be severe, and is an unconscious expression of a woman's sexual anxiety. When severe it can appear there is no opening to the vagina, but a history of a normal menstrual flow will exclude the possibility of a congenital deformity. Sometimes dilators are used to encourage a woman to 'stretch herself', but this can reinforce the idea that the genitals should not be touched. However the experience of learning to use a contraceptive cap or a dilator may help her to understand the flexibility and stretchiness of her vagina.

If first attempts at intercourse have been painful, the fear of pain then leads to adductor spasm and tension, which makes it impossible to examine the vagina. Once the woman can accept examination, it is extremely rare to find a hymenal ring which cannot be stretched by gentle pressure from the fingers.

To learn to explore the vagina with her own fingers can be helpful, not only with regard to the size of the introitus, but also allowing an exploration of her ideas about touching herself, the way the vagina is formed, and the implications of penetration. We have seen that Nurse C was able to enjoy intercourse once she had been able to part with the fantasy she had about her vagina. When a patient starts to describe the way she thinks of herself, it is important that the doctor should listen carefully and uncritically, respecting and not ridiculing the ideas which are offered, so that the patient can gradually replace the fantasy with reality.

Twelve years of marriage elapsed before Mr and Mrs G decided they would like a child. Mrs G went to the GP, who told her there was no treatment for her complaint, that intercourse was impossible. Determined to start a family, Mrs G made enquiries at the public library, and referred herself to the clinic. She attended alone, telling the doctor in great distress of her longing to conceive. 'It's all my fault; I have a block. I just can't let him inside.' When they were first married Mrs G had clammed up every time he had attempted penetration, although when they were engaged and content to accept the strict family prohibition on pre-marital sex, she had longed to make love. She tried to relax, but it was useless. They gave up attempting penetration, and over the years they had enjoyed sexual pleasure in a variety of ways, including oral intercourse, and both had been able to have a climax. It was only when they wanted a child that the problem resurfaced.

The doctor suggested an examination might help in understanding the difficulty. Mrs G took a long time to undress, then lay on the couch with her knees drawn together, looking very apprehensive. When the doctor remarked on her anxiety, she replied that she thought it would hurt. 'So it must be delicate', said the doctor. 'I will stop as soon as you say.' Mrs G looked relieved, and was surprised that it did not hurt when the doctor was able to insert a finger. Then she talked of her fear of pain, and as she did so the doctor was able to feel the tightening of the vagina. It gripped his finger, and he could show her how the fear had caused the pain. There was a long pause while she thought about this, then the doctor suggested she should feel what it was like for herself; she hesitated, then inserted the tip of her finger, looking surprised when it slipped in easily.

The following week Mrs G got on the couch with alacrity, and when the doctor was examining her she was able to talk, tentatively, about her image of the vagina; that it was a narrow, rigid tube which would split and burst on penetration, with severe pain and bleeding. With such an unacknowledged thought it was only reasonable to prevent penetration. Having listened carefully, and by encouraging self-exploration the doctor was able to help her to compare the reality of her vagina with the fantasy. At the next appointment the couple had consummated their marriage, and soon Mrs G was pregnant.

It was the use of the thoughts and feelings expressed during the vaginal examination that made it possible to resolve Mrs G's difficulty in a comparatively short time. Listening to patients in this way, one hears many descriptions of the vagina and the hymen which imply that penetration will be painful and bloody. It is important to be able to understand the specific fantasy of the patient, and not to try to fit the fantasy to the patient.

Sometimes there is confusion as to the functions of that area of the body. One woman came back to the clinic looking pleased and relieved when she had used a tampon for the first time. She had been amazed to find that when she had passed water the tampon was not wet! In this way she had been able to learn of the separation of the vagina and the bladder, and now felt free to use the vagina for its proper purpose. This fantasy may arise from the biological cloaca found in some animals.

> Mrs H was referred from a sex therapy clinic that used Master's and Johnson's techniques because she could not bear to be touched, and so was unable to follow the programme. She said she had been given glass dilators to use, but found the idea abhorrent. Offered an examination, she showed the doctor her thoughts by saying, 'I don't know how you can bear to do that.' When this had been discussed, she agreed to have an examination, although she lay on the couch with her nose wrinkled in disgust. There was no vaginismus; just an air of profound distaste. During a number of visits, the vaginal examination was used to enable her to express her feelings that the vagnia was unnatural, dirty, connected with excretion, and that sperm were nasty and smelled! Sharing these thoughts with the doctor helped to make them less prohibitive. Progress was erratic; Mrs H would show courage in touching and thinking about this 'nasty place' and then relapse and talk of the 'raw wound'. Suddenly, she came back after the Christmas holiday to say she could go to bed without dreading it; that she could accept the doctor, her husband's fingers, and finally his penis as part of life. She added that previously they had no visitors in their flat, but now they were enjoying entertaining their friends!

The symbolic meanings of the vaginal examination have been described (Tunnadine, 1970). Often a patient will talk about the way she feels about her house – the need for privacy or lack of it, the messiness, and her mother's influence in it – and sometimes it is possible for the doctor to make a comparison with this and the way the patient feels about intercourse in terms of the patient's feelings as a whole person.

COUPLES OR SINGLES

At the first visit the doctor can only examine whoever attends the consultation, bearing in mind that a couple may attend together, not because they have chosen to, but because the referring agency thought that all sexual therapy must be with both partners. If it is considered that the difficulty is primarily intrapersonal, that is, the root of the problem lies in the patient's inner world, then this work can only be done with the individual on their own. When the difficulty is interpersonal, within the relationship, then they may be seen as a couple so the events of the consultation can be used (Draper, 1983).

Women who attend alone for treatment have been shown to achieve twice the consummation rate of those who attend as couples throughout (Bramley *et al.*, 1983), demonstrating the value of allowing the exploration of half-hidden thoughts in private. The doctor may therefore choose to work with the partners separately. In the following case, working with the woman alone provided an opportunity to explore her feelings and her body together.

> Mr and Mrs J were referred to the clinic by a gynaecologist, who wrote that he had performed a plastic enlargement of the vagina with the intention of using dilators later. He had chosen a mechanical approach because Mrs J already had been treated by two psychiatrists for long-standing non-consummation.
>
> At the first consultation, Mr J was bluff and over-confident, while Mrs J sat and glowered. With encouragement, however, she was able to give a graphic description of her experience when she 'came to' after the operation, which she had expected to resolve all her troubles. Her mother was sitting beside her, and she gradually became aware of something strange sticking out between her legs, which made her feel both embarrassed and uncomfortable. The nurse came and explained that it was a dilator. The nurse took it out, but the mucosa had dried, and the removal was painful and made her feel sick. Three weeks later she tried to use the dilator herself, as instructed, but it was 'horrible!' Since then several doctors had been unable to examine her, and an attempt to make love when deliberately drunk had failed.
>
> Although somewhat daunted by her 'impenetrability' and the way it had been increased by repeated therapeutic failures, the doctor was impressed by the

strength of Mrs J's persistent search for help. She and her husband were now living apart, and the doctor, thinking it was important to work with Mrs J's feelings about herself, arranged to see her alone. Mr J came on his own once to discuss his anxieties, but he then decided to prove he was 'all right' by having a girlfriend.

At first it was necessary to allow Mrs J to work through repeatedly the anger, resentment, and depression caused by her failed treatments. It was important to allow her knowingly to be in control of the examination, starting with just touching the perineum. Significantly, being 'in touch' with the vagina also allowed her to tell the doctor they had both enjoyed heavy petting and oral sex, when she easily had a climax. When she talked of her home, Mrs J said sex was never discussed, and her husband had to 'tell her about it' on her wedding night; later she said she thought she had heard her parents having sex when there had been dreadful rows. Because she trusted the doctor Mrs J confided she thought her vagina was 'too small to allow anything in; tapering, delicate, a narrow tube all filled up.' With the doctor's help she was able to find the reality of her own vagina.

It took a number of visits before Mrs J was able to lose her vaginismus. Meanwhile, she had several tense and difficult meetings with her husband. Once the examination became relaxed, the doctor decided to make a distant appointment so there was no pressure to perform. Two months later she came back and said they had 'done it'; the first few times she just lay there and felt nothing, but now, she said laughing, 'I just can't believe the difficulty.'

This couple managed to find individual help; the woman from her doctor and presumably the husband from his girlfriend, and they were then able to re-establish the relationship. It is not always possible to achieve such a happy outcome. Mrs J was persistent in her attendance, but others will be ambivalent, keeping some appointments and missing others and then re-booking and failing to turn up – unable to co-operate in their treatment in a way that would lead to a resolution of their problem.

Some couples choose each other unconsciously, for complimentary sexual difficulties. The woman who complains of non-consummation will often describe her partner as 'kind and gentle'. It often happens that when she has overcome her fears of penetration he becomes temporarily impotent, revealing that he too had sexual anxieties which need help. When only one member of a couple seeks treatment, the doctor may have to reconcile himself to the fact that an individual may be helped to mature at the expense of the partnership, which may later break up.

Sometimes the sexual problem is part of a more widespread psychological problem, and therefore a brief psychosomatic approach is unsuitable.

> One day Mrs K became very upset at the family planning clinic, which she had attended for the past 10 years. She told the doctor that her father had died recently. The doctor made a sympathetic response, and she went on to whisper that she only came to the clinic for the Pill because she had suffered from severe dysmenorrhoea, and that her marriage had never been consummated. The doctor offered her an appointment at the psychosexual problem clinic, where there would be more time to talk, and this was accepted. Mrs K kept several appointments, and was always upset, talking of her father's death and her dreams of him. Everything she had done in her life – her academic achievements, her senior job in the Civil Service, had been for him. She did not think she had done anything just for herself. When the doctor suggested an examination, she refused. By now she had given up her job. She started talking to the doctor about some embroideries she was planning, using wartime images of destruction. The doctor grew anxious that any attempt to work towards consummation was going to upset Mrs K's fragile psychological equilibrium. More regular psychotherapy was offered and declined. After full discussion, and by mutual consent, it was agreed 'to let sleeping dogs lie', and Mrs K ceased to attend. Her sexual problem was only a small part of the greater difficulty of maturation.

The inability to achieve intercourse is only a symptom; behind it there is always some barrier or wall that prevents full penetration in sexual intercourse. This barrier can represent a continuum of difficulty. At one extreme there are women such a Mrs G who are able to enjoy sexual feelings and have a climax, and in whom the difficulty is confined to a fantasy about genital organs and the perils of the first act of intercourse. At the other extreme are those who cannot accept themselves as sexual people. Most lie in the centre of the continuum. They have difficulties not only in the area of genital fantasy and of not being in control, but also in acceptance of their sexuality and in maturation and separation from their parents.

By using the 'tools of our trade' – the psychosomatic vaginal examination and the insights gained through the doctor/paient relationship in successive consultations – we can often work towards a satisfactory outcome. The barrier, perceptible in the consultation, then can be removed, brick by brick, through interpretations of the events in the here and now. Putting a woman in touch with her sexuality in this way can cause such a tranformation in her general manner that she gains confidence in all aspects of her life.

REFERENCES

Bramley, H. M., Brown, J., Draper K. C. and Kilvington, J. (1981) Brief psychosomatic therapy for consummation of marriage. *Br. J. Obs. Gynae.*, 88, 819–24.

Bramley, H. M., Brown, J., Draper, K. C. and Kilvington, J. (1983) Non-consummation of marriage treated by members of the Institute of Psychosexual Medicine: a prospective study. *Br. J. Obs. Gynae.*, 90, 908–13.

Draper, K. C. (1983) Working as a co-therapist, in *Practice of Psychosexual Medicine* (Ed. K. C. Draper), J. Libbey, London.

Rodwell, L. (1987) A couple unjoined in matrimony. *The Independent*, 7 July, p. 13.

Tunnadine, L. P. D. (1970) *Contraception and Sexual Life*, Tavistock Publications, London.

Valins, L. (1988) *Vaginismus: Understanding and Overcoming Blocks to Intercourse*, Ashgrove Press, Bath.

8

Problems with orgasm

Joan Coombs

SUMMARY

- Problems with technique and communication
- Orgasm and sexual abuse
- The fear of letting go
- Anorgasmia and the menopause
- Bereavement

Most doctors when confronted by a patient complaining of difficulties with orgasm feel dismayed and sometimes anxious.

The orgasm is a mysterious event, particularly in females. Many attempts, medical and literary, have been made to define it. John Bancroft (1983) wrote, 'It is difficult to define because it is such a subjective experience occurring often at a time when one's powers of observation are impaired if not suspended.'

For men, the experience is marked visually by ejaculation. Sometimes impairment of the internal bladder sphincter may result in retrograde ejaculation. The seminal fluid is driven back into the bladder and the man may be disappointed to experience the sensations of orgasm without evidence of it. For females the experience is apparently more varied. Masters and Johnson (1966) describe it as, 'a psychophysiologic experience occurring within and made meaningful by a context of psychosocial influence. Physiologically it is a brief episode of physical release from the vasocongestive and myotonic increment developed in response to sexual stimuli.'

The *Oxford Concise Dictionary* defines orgasm as violent excitement, rage, paroxysm. The height of venereal excitement in coition. Sigmund Freud reported a difference between the 'clitoral orgasm' and the 'vaginal orgasm', interpreting the former as the juvenile version. Masters and Johnson conducted a series of investigations involving a group of women who were motivated and able to perform sexually under laboratory conditions. They deduced that 'When any woman experiences orgasmic response to effective sexual stimulation the vagina and clitoris react in consistent physiologic patterns. Thus clitoral and vaginal orgasms are not separate biologic entities.' In other words, excitement is excitement is excitement. It is interesting that Freud did not feel constrained to compare the quality of the male orgasm in the presence or absence of the vagina.

One hundred years after Freud, Dr Prudence Tunnadine (1970) writes on orgasm with the penis in the vagina: 'The togetherness, mutual abandonment of control systems, the emotional acceptance of the penis and all it implies in terms of the man, and of the vagina and all that it implies in terms of the woman, makes this a unique experience that is not mimicked emotionally by mutual masturbation however loving. It is emotionally more difficult for many people and many who cannot achieve it are in no doubt as to its importance or as to the difference.'

The importance of this wish for togetherness and happiness through perfect sex is exploited commercially. Advertising plays on a whole range of emotions – the desire for status, the desire to look good, the desire to be a good mother, the desire for things to be as they used to be in those past golden days mellowed by hindsight. The USP – the Unique Selling Proposition – implies that use of the product will bring happiness. Among the dreams of happiness are those of perfect sexual experience. Much sexual activity that is depicted on television and in films and magazines involves the ultimate in sexual performance. Couples copulate with the maximum arousal, often with the minimum of preludes. Orgasms are achieved by penetration and are simultaneous. These are the fantasies of the advertising men and the script writers, and represent their wishes and beliefs about human sexuality.

Real life is mundane and prosaic, and for some the nearness to perfection is something that happens rarely.

The public are surrounded by sexual awareness. Few people are unaffected by the brave talk and bragging of others. Our own anxieties make us quake and feel diminished by comparison. Perhaps one of the most important things a doctor can do is to help the patient to examine those expectations of sex that are appropriate, and those that are not. Listening to what the patient has to say may help the doctor to understand better. All the while, the doctor has to contend with his or her own feelings of inadequacy concerning 'the trouble with orgasm'. 'Why didn't they teach me better in medical school?', 'What is the treatment for anorgasmia?' may be the deafening lament. The truth is that anorgasmia is not an illness but a presenting symptom to alert the doctor's attention. Patients offer doctors 'visiting cards' or present them with 'tickets of entry'. The true reason for the consultation may not be revealed until the patient says on the point of leaving, 'Oh, by the way, doctor'.

PROBLEMS WITH TECHNIQUE AND COMMUNICATION

Andrea, aged 23, came to see her GP for treatment for her persisting dyspepsia and weight gain. She had started the combined oral contraceptive pill shortly before her marriage to Bill nearly two years ago. Andrea was happy with her new lifestyle and loved her husband. She enjoyed cooking for him but always overestimated their needs. However, she couldn't bear waste and was apt to eat the surplus food. The patient's diagnosis was that the obesity was due to the Pill. The doctor was unwilling to accept this, and listened to what else the patient had to say. The discussion between them led to better understanding of the weight problem and dyspepsia.

The doctor felt the consultation was over, and the patient stood up to go. Then she sat down looking distressed. 'There's another problem too. I don't have an organism (sic) – a climax. I love being with Bill and I do get excited, but as soon as I think I might feel it, it goes away. Bill is getting very cross about it and said I need a doctor.' The doctor felt overwhelmed, and was aware of the people yet to be seen in the waiting-room. The pressure on the doctor was intense. The doctor said, 'We can't discuss this quickly with all the other patients waiting. Would you like to come back and see me again when we can discuss the problem without this feeling of pressure?'

Two subsequent consultations led to greater understanding of the troubles. The patient had complained that she did not have an 'organism' with sex with her husband. The *Oxford Concise Dictionary* defines 'organism' as, 'Organized body with connected interdependent parts sharing common life.' This was a very appropriate description of Andrea's hopes of her marriage with Bill. They had not lived together prior to their marriage. There had been little pressure on them during their sexual courtship. They made love when they felt like it, in relative privacy and unhampered by parental disapproval. The atmosphere between the two of them was highly charged, and it was understood how much they meant to each other, although little was said. In many ways they were making love to the fantasy partners each had dreamed about. Preludes were inappropriate as sexual tension had been building up for years in anticipation. Sex was delightful, and Andrea was orgasmic with penetration. They looked forward to better things.

After their marriage, the reality of their life together was not so easy. Both expected Andrea to carry on where Bill's mother had left off in terms of care of the household and of his domestic needs. Andrea tried to conform, and suppressed her feelings of irritation and disappointment with Bill, who had previously been her ideal man. It was with difficulty that she shared her anger with the doctor. When it came to sex, Bill was apt to approach rapidly with no more preludes than before. Whereas before she was delighted to welcome him, she found it difficult when she was feeling resentful. Bill's speedy approach and premature penetration was usually followed by rapid ejaculation. Their awareness of her disappointment made him retreat into feigned sleep, but with a resolution to do better next time.

Andrea explained there was never enough time for

her to become aroused. Now she was beginning to prevent arousal by thinking of shopping lists and tomor-
row's programme in an attempt to insulate herself from
the expectation of her husband's disappointing love-
making. To make matters worse, he saw her frigidity as
her problem, which required medical treatment; he did
not see it as a stalemate to which he contributed – he
dared not. Andrea felt powerless and used. The only
weapon she truly owned in this losing battle of the sexes
was her failure to provide the desired orgasm. This was
the only way she could render him less than cocksure.
In spite of Andrea's original description of how much
she loved her husband, her anger and exasperation with
him became apparent. The doctor noticed it, but at the
same time did not see Bill as the villain. She shared
with Andrea the comment that he probably was not
pleased with his own sexual performance. She also
noted that as long as the disappointment continued he
would continue to see Andrea as unsatisfiable and
threatening.

The basic problem between the couple was failure of communication. They were like two closed books to each other, each
containing wishes of oneness, 'interdependent parts sharing a
common life', but without the skill to build on their wishful thinking with verbal understanding.

Because of the emphasis on sexual performance that assails the
individual from the media and from gossip and social intercourse,
many people consider the woman who does not have a climax as
abnormal. Often these same people are ignorant of the fact that
the clitoris is as important an organ as the penis for satisfying
intercourse.

A man is incapable of penetration and completing intravaginal
intercourse without sexual excitement leading to engorgement of
the spongy tissues and erection. Females are capable of receiving
penetration and accepting intercourse without any stimulation or
arousal. Needless to say, such intercourse is not a sexual pleasure,
but many woman have done and still do simulate pleasure so as
to protect self-esteem, either that of their partner or their own.
Fairburn, Dickerson, and Greenwood (1983) comment, 'It is not
common knowledge that most women require clitoral stimulation
if they are to reach orgasm'.

For Andrea such stimulation had not been necessary in the highly charged atmosphere of their pre-marital love-making. Faced with the reality of having to contain negative as well as positive feelings towards her husband, she did not become aroused so spontaneously and more foreplay was necessary. After talking to the doctor she was able to communicate more of her physical needs to her husband, as well as dealing more directly with her angry feelings, which were inhibiting her sexual arousal.

The doctor's time invested in the early marriage of this couple was not wasted. Although the husband was not seen at this stage by the doctor, he began to feel safer in his wife's company, and they learned pace and pleasure in their love-making.

Talking and thinking in the doctor's company helped Andrea talk and develop understanding within the marriage. Not only was the psychosexual problem helped, but the couple developed skills in resolving other conflicts.

ORGASM AND SEXUAL ABUSE

The next psychosexual problem appeared to present in a similar way.

Caroline was in her mid-20s, and came to see the doctor for a repeat prescription for her combined contraceptive pill. She had been sharing a home with David for nearly three years. She presented her problem directly: 'Doctor, please can you help me, there's a problem with sex and I never get a climax.'

Once again the doctor was in a difficult spot. There was no quick answer and other patients were waiting. Traditional responses are recognizable to all doctors. To use insights gained from the doctor's previous case would have been inappropriate. 'You need to talk more. Let genital caressing continue after his premature ejaculation. Be patient, it will improve. Shall we change your pill?' All of these responses would have been inappropriate, as the problem had not yet been examined. They would have served to get the patient out of the room. The reassurance might have comforted the doctor, but certainly not the patient. In truth, the cases, although presenting in a similar way, were quite different. Later the doctor understood.

Caroline had been briefly happy having sex with David

but now it was terrible. She could not respond in any way. The doctor let her talk and the story came pouring out. Caroline was the only daughter of a family of five children. Both her parents had been unhappily married before, and then were unhappily married to each other. Caroline's younger two brothers were both conceived accidentally as the couple used no efficient method of birth control. When the youngest was born, Caroline's parents took to separate bedrooms. Caroline and her mother worked full-time, and Caroline helped with the shopping, cooking, and cleaning. Her father worked shifts.

Caroline was 'daddy's girl' and he was the one person who showed her love and affection. There was much cuddling, which she enjoyed. They kept it secret, and the cuddling developed into genital fondling. At this point Caroline became fearful and aware that what was happening was wrong. She felt helpless and alone. She was unable to discuss it with her mother. Caroline explained her isolation. She felt orphaned. She had no mother who she was able to relate to. She had longed for fatherly tenderness, love, and protection and had felt orphaned by her father's passion and preoccupation with sex. She felt trapped by the secrecy. She described her way of coping with life, which was to separate herself from the experience of what was happening. Full intercourse took place, but Caroline would pretend to herself that she was part of the wall alongside the bed.

The doctor's feelings were of overwhelming concern for this child-woman. The urge to become a mothering doctor was strong. With no prompting the story went on.

Caroline grew up feeling alone, different, unlovable, and, worst of all, dirty and guilty. When she met David and he loved her she found delight and pleasure in herself. She dared not tell him of her past in case he rejected her in disgust. David badly wanted to marry. He wanted a wife, home, and children, but most of all he wanted Caroline and to be with her. Caroline agreed to live with him, but she would not marry him: her parents' marriages had been unhappy traps, and she did not want to be trapped ever again. She had a need to be in charge of herself and her world, and never to surrender to the position of victim again.

During the consultations the doctor was to feel Caroline's power and control. It was difficult for Caroline to perceive any of the doctor's comments or interpretations. Whenever the doctor spoke, Caroline would talk against her. The story continued.

During their early courtship, when their longing for each other was intense, they would make love frequently. However, Caroline was always in charge, and would never surrender completely to her sexual excitement. She had a great need to say no, and for it to be accepted. David complied.

When they had been living together for a year or so, they found that the contract negotiations of 'who does what' in the house were difficult to resolve. They both worked full-time. After work Caroline would do most of the domestic work while David watched TV. She was too busy to go to the pub with him, so he took up snooker. By bedtime she felt helpless, angry, and used. She was less and less able to respond to David as she had used to do. Gradually, she began to vent her anger, at first punishing him with her passive, silent, long-suffering sexual response, later forcing rows, swearing at him, and beating him with her fists. The doctor said perhaps this was some of the anger she had felt for her father, but had not expressed. Caroline agreed she used David as the whipping-boy. When she closed her eyes during love-making it seemed as if it was her father, and not David.

Gradually, Caroline worked through her need to recount everything. She felt much relief from the telling of the tale. Her lifelong fear that if the truth were known she would be totally abandoned led her to expect the doctor to reject her. The doctor did not reject her, but went on listening and learning.

The patient arranged a joint consultation, though not at the doctor's suggestion, and brought David with her. He was awkward, shy, and not good with words. In spite of this, he was apparently pleased to be in the doctor's company, and an air of anticipation preceded their talk. Two weeks previously Caroline had told David of her

past. His first reaction had been one of relief. He had
said, 'I'm so glad. I thought you were rejecting me
because I was no good.' The surprise and irony of his
reaction led to some merriment. They were kindred spir-
its after all.

And so the saga went on. Once Caroline and David were able to
function honestly as a couple they had the basis on which to build
trust and understanding into their relationship. Caroline did not
become orgasmic – she did not want to go that far yet – but
they were content with their love-making, which became a shared
pleasure and excitement again.

The doctor's function had been as the non-judging listener.
By resisting the pressure to mother this orphaned child she had
refrained from infantilizing her, and had treated her as an adult
with the potential for a satisfying sexual life. In time, this was
how Caroline came to see herself – not damaged and scarred for
life. The sexual complaint of anorgasmia had been the patient's
visiting card, the token that had alerted the doctor's attention to
the underlying trouble.

Many such patients, who struggle with a sense of defilement
and guilt resulting from childhood sexual activity feel that in some
way they are maimed or changed genitally. While they fear the
genital examination, they can be greatly reassured by it. Often
the doctor is unaware of the patient's secret fears and fantasies,
and yet should remain sensitive to the patient's perception of the
genital examination, which is in effect a psychosomatic event.
Doctors should be alert to the possible misinterpretation of comments about these 'private parts'. It is not unknown for a casual
remark unwittingly made to reinforce a patient's worst fears
regarding size and dirtiness.

Often girls who have experienced sexual activity during childhood – whether as a pleasure or as the recipient of another's
needs – have persisting feelings of guilt, wretchedness, and a need
to keep these feelings private. Because they are the life-long
custodians of secrets, and never risk revelation, they must keep
control at all times. They guard their emanations; they resist
anaesthetics; they prevent that ultimate letting go – the experience
of orgasm – lest the secret be revealed.

Today, the disclosure or revelation of childhood sexual activity
is more acceptable than in the past. We are at the frontiers of
understanding; there is a hope that disclosure is therapeutic, but

what follows revelation is still a mystery. Further study will enlighten us as to whether disclosure allows individuals to escape the hauntings from the past, leaving them free to develop their emotional lives, and free to celebrate their own sexuality in orgasm.

Sometimes girls who have been involved sexually with an adult during childhood grow to avoid sexual activity during adult life. Not all early experiences are violent and demanding. If the child's lover was gentle and tender, it is likely that the child was sexually responsive; pleasure may have been part of her sexual experience. Social awareness may develop only after these events, at which time the child learns to detest her pleasure and her part in the seduction. Such girls commonly inhibit their natural sexual responses, finding them disgusting.

THE FEAR OF LETTING GO

Being orgasmic has to do with the letting go of control. One of the earliest lessons in life is that associated with toilet training and gaining control of the bladder and anal sphincters. We learn that we are loveable when we are clean and dry. We may learn that we are not loveable when we are wet and dirty and not controlling this part of our body.

Elaine took her six-month-old daughter to the doctor because she had been feverish and restless with a troublesome cough. The doctor examined the child and prescribed, but noticed that Elaine looked unhappy. She asked her how she was, and although Elaine was at the door the doctor asked her to sit down. She did so and wept. Everything was wrong: the birth had been awful. She had studied all the books, been to all the classes, and had a plan in her head as to how it would go, but it hadn't been a bit as she'd planned. It was more painful than she had expected. She cried and moaned and asked for an epidural after all, but it was too late as things were going too fast. She had planned not to have an episiotomy, but did. Elaine said she felt ashamed of her performance, and unhappy that Frank, her husband, had been disappointed too.

After the birth she had difficulty with her bladder and

had to have a catheter. Her stitches were painful and her bowels were difficult. Breast feeding was nothing like she expected, and she had given up and put the baby on the bottle.

Life with the baby was chaotic; she had always been so organized before, with her responsible job and the lovely home that she and Frank had made together. Suddenly everything was in total disorder – no routine and no pleasure. She had been aware that Frank felt shut out by her preoccupation with the baby. She wanted to respond when he made love to her, but she could not. She used to reach a climax often before the baby was born, but it had not happened once since the birth.

The doctor and Elaine talked that day and again later. The doctor discovered that all her life Elaine had tried to be in control. She was the eldest of her mother's five children, and had always been the grown-up, sensible one, the 'little mother' who helped her mother. She bitterly resented being 'out of control' in her labour, and out of control with her bladder and bowels, feeling guilty about what she considered to be a 'bad' performance. She felt she was not being a good enough mother to her little daughter. She did not feel worthy enough to enjoy love-making, and was out of touch with her pleasure. In fact, her stitches had not hurt for long, but she found herself preoccupied with her baby. Even when the baby was asleep Elaine would keep vigil; she could not allow sexual excitement and orgasm as it would interrupt this. The doctor also learned that Elaine was not able to reconcile being a mother with being a sexual woman. As a child she had felt that mothers should be mothers. She found her own mother's sexuality deeply shocking, and had resented it.

Gradually, Elaine came to terms with these contributing factors and rediscovered peace of mind and pleasure in her relationship with Frank. She also rediscovered her capacity for orgasm once the guilt and disappointment had faded.

There are many factors that may contribute to post-natal anorgasmia. Apart from the doubt about whether mothers should be sexual or not, there is often much less opportunity for love-making. Life is busier and more tiring than it used to be. A young baby is a very demanding person, and most parents recognize what good contraceptive agents babies and small children are by always keeping parents apart. Apart from perineal discomfort and breast activity in the lactating mother, there are often bodily changes, albeit temporary, which may undermine sexual confidence. The woman who feels she has lost her girlish figure and has become matronly often feels that sexiness has gone too.

Just as the girl has ambitions for herself as a new mother, she also has hopes for her partner as the ideal father. If he behaves badly in the labour ward, or is not there when she needs him she will resent it. If he behaves badly and is jealous of the attention the baby gets she will reward him with her sexual apathy.

ANORGASMIA AND THE MENOPAUSE

Although the physical problems of vaginal dryness at the time of the menopause can be relieved by hormone replacement therapy, this does not always solve the problem.

Mary went to her doctor complaining of a total lack of interest in sex. He referred her to a psychosexual clinic with the following letter: 'I have seen Mary on several occasions. She is 52 and I started her on hormone replacement therapy. Vaginal examination revealed a healthy vaginal mucosa. She tells me she has no problems with vaginal dryness. Her hot flushes have settled but she remains totally disinterested in sex with her husband. They are both deeply unhappy; perhaps something can be done.'

Mary and her husband came together for their first session. Mary was a tall, dignified woman, beautifully dressed, quiet and polite. Her husband was unhappy and tense. During the conversation they both seemed to feel hopeless, and the doctor began to feel unhappy too. They talked about their happy 25-year marriage together. Both had wanted children, and they had had two, who were now grown up and gone from home. Mary had been an only child, and it was only with difficulty that she had broken free of the parental home. To start with sex had been very difficult. She had been passive and frightened, and her husband had been afraid of hurting her. In spite of this they had developed a happy sexual life together. When they first became parents there were difficulties, but once again things improved and they took it for granted that sex was a continuing blessing.

The doctor felt she was at a wake, talking over old times and lamenting death. She asked Mary what she felt about her menopause. Her periods had stopped two years ago. She was sad but not excessively so, the hot flushes bearable and not intense. The doctor felt something was missing, and wondered why the problem had started now.

Mary related how her mother had begun to decline when her father died three years ago. She was unhappy living alone and longed to live with her daughter. Once her mother had moved in, Mary's old difficulties came flooding back. She became intensely aware of her mother, and also of her disapproval of sexuality. She worried about being overheard in their bedroom, and avoided any sign of affection between her and her husband, feeling they were being observed by her mother. She felt angry with her mother, but also guilty about having these feelings.

Mary's capacity to celebrate her own sexuality completely vanished. Without arousal she found intercourse an ordeal and a trial. She could not remember when she last experienced a climax. She talked at length about how she had felt her mother to be forbidding of her daughter's sexuality when she was young and how her present predicament echoed these feelings; her feelings of guilt and anger interfered with her ability to let go to the sex and excitement.

Mary was pleased with the conversation and wanted another appointment. However, she did not come, and instead wrote saying that it was not necessary: things were much better and they were much happier. Had they put her mother in a home, or was Mary claiming sex for herself? The doctor was left puzzling.

This woman's feelings of guilt about her anger at her mother made it difficult for her to discuss the problem with her family doctor. The doctor assumed the problems were menopausal, and was bewildered when HRT did not cure the unhappiness.

BEREAVEMENT

Bereavement commonly affects sexual functioning and inhibits orgasm. Many who are bereaved feel personal pleasure is inappropriate during mourning; it somehow seems improper to enjoy anything when one is preoccupied with loss. The experience of mourning has to do with the constant remembering of the lost one. Arousal and orgasm have something to do with the forgetting of the outside world, and are often not permitted by those who mourn.

Anger is part of mourning. Why did it happen? Why me? Such anger has to be worked through before it can be laid aside. Sometimes the fear of being overwhelmed by grief can inhibit the abandonment and vulnerability necessary for orgasm.

Bereavement is not only for the loss of a loved person. It also can be for the loss of self-esteem and impairment of body-image. Mastectomy, colostomy, sterilization, cancer, disfigurements and many other conditions can all bring loss of sexual confidence. Infertility, and the recurring death of hope that each menstrual period brings is a powerful inhibition of sexual arousal and climax (p. 180). Finally, the death of trust that follows betrayal or adultery is often felt as a numbing bereavement.

Gloria and Harry had been married for many years. They lived rather dull, monotonous lives, and their only daughter worked abroad. Sex had never been exciting, but Gloria enjoyed Harry's approaches. She never gave any signs of pleasure: she had learned at her mother's knee that nice girls are passive and leave it up to the men. Harry was weary of this and longed for excitement. At work he welcomed the enthusiasm of a new typist, and their friendship fast developed into a sexual passion. To ease his guilt, Harry confessed to his wife. She was devastated by his confession, but galvanized into sexual hunger for him – a kind of competitive response. For the first time in her life she had a climax. The deterioration of trust and confidence between them overwhelmed them both. Soon Gloria found that her despair prevented any arousal or pleasure from the ritual that their intercourse had become.

Although failure to achieve orgasm is not a treatable illness in the usual sense, it is a very important symptom. The causes are many.

Listening to the patient will help the doctor to learn what factors are contributing, whether they are unrealistic expectations, poor sexual technique, or a fear of letting go. It follows that the doctor's response may be just as varied as the factors producing the symptom. If poor sexual technique is the problem, the doctor's response is clear, but rarely are things as simple as telling the patient what to do, or giving the patient 'permission' to do this or that. Nor is it helpful to tell a patient to 'let go' if not being able to let go is the problem.

Like the patient, the harder the doctor attempts to reach the apple, the more the apple remains out of reach. Anorgasmia is not a symptom that responds to treatment in the traditional sense. Sensitive listening encourages the patient to understand 'why now', to discuss where the block comes from, in the past or in the here and now. Discussion helps the patient to recognize her own part in resolving the problem. It is not the doctor's responsibility; ultimately it is the woman herself who prevents the orgasmic experience, and ultimately she is the one who permits it.

REFERENCES

Bancroft, J. (1989) *Human Sexuality and its Problems*, 2nd edn, Churchill Livingstone, Edinburgh, p. 77.

Fairburn, C., Dickerson, M. and Greenwood, J. (1983) *Sexual Problems and their Management*, Churchill Livingstone, Edinburgh.

Masters, W. and Johnson, V. (1966) *Human Sexual Response*, Little, Brown & Company, Boston, Ch. 9.

Tunnadine, P. (1970) *Contraception and Sexual Life*, Tavistock Publications, London.

9

Loss of libido

Rosemarie Lincoln

SUMMARY

- Diagnosis
- Depression
- Relationship problems
- Anger behind the need to please
- Mourning
- Post-natal disturbance
- Self-punishment or control
- The therapeutic encounter

Doctors usually feel rather gloomy when presented with the very common problem of loss of interest in sex. Perhaps it is symbolic of the symptom that it can be mentioned with a throwaway line such as, 'I suppose I'm just bored with sex now that I'm 40 and have been married a long time,' or, 'I don't seem to feel much like making love any more. Do you think it's due to the Pill?' Sometimes there may be a more emphatic approach, such as, 'I can't bear my husband to touch me nowadays.'

The atmosphere of withdrawal behind barriers can be felt in the doctor/patient relationship, and understanding the cause of

Source: *The Practitioner*, Vol. 233, pp. 1315–18, 1989.

Loss of libido

those barriers is the key to the diagnosis. There are several questions the doctor should ask himself. Is this true loss of libido, or has it always been so? Primary lack of sexual libido, which in the woman would be called frigidity, is the result of difficulty in psychosexual development and may result from early childhood emotional deprivation. Experiences of child sexual abuse, or rape in adolescence may hinder normal sexual libidinal maturation. Is this patient really wanting help for him-/herself? Someone who is attending to placate or to blame the partner is really a non-patient, with very little motivation for change. The doctor may even be tempted to send for the partner, which is seldom as helpful as working with the partner who has presented. If the symptom is of long duration, why has the complaint been made now? Is it that a life event has triggered the request for help, or is there a fear of the break-up of the marriage?

DIAGNOSIS

The essential task in psychosexual medicine, as in all medicine, is to try and make an accurate diagnosis before treatment – but therein lies considerable difficulty for the doctor. In this sensitive and anxiety-laden area the defences for most people are strong. Our psyche protects us from pain, and direct questioning produces answers that may be far from the truth. To diagnose the problem, the doctor has to find a way around the defences, which may present as the total idealization of the relationship, or the denial of bad feelings about a life event, in terms such as, 'Of course, it was just one of those things, and other people have far more to put up with.' Although each person's problem is unique and has to be studied carefully, some common aetiological factors emerge that may change the sexual libido. The loss may be associated with a general depression; anger in response to relationship difficulties; mourning; post-natal emotional disturbance due to events experienced during pregnancy and delivery; echoes from childhood; relationship difficulties; or with self-punishment after such events as termination of pregnancy or sexual promiscuity.

DEPRESSION

A characteristic feature of depression is the loss of interest in many aspects of life, with the absence of joy and excitement. It is therefore not surprising that sexual libido is also affected. Unfortunately, this will often increase the depression because the deterioration of communication with the partner contributes further to the internalized anger. In both men and women a change of libido can be attributed to the many causes of depression, such as redundancy, job failure, ageing, retirement, post-natal problems, infertility, mourning, rejection, and so on. The capacity to reach orgasm may be affected as well as the mood and the appetite for sexual pleasure.

The following case-history describes a man who became angry because his plans in his job did not work out as he had hoped. His mood was depressed and affected his sexual libido, especially as he could not share his frustration with his wife.

A good-looking, slim and articulate man of about 38 sought help because he had not felt in the mood for making love with his wife for about a year. If he did so, really to please her, his potency was often unreliable and caused more distress. The quality of their sexual life had previously been mutually rewarding, and the couple could not understand what had gone wrong. Their life was materially comfortable, with no financial worries and a very nice house, to which the wife devoted her time and to caring for their twin boys of eight. It was difficult to find any factors in the man's life that might affect his sexual interest, but, in accordance with the maxim that if the doctor waits long enough the patient will tell him the problem, he eventually began to describe his (well-defended) unhappiness at work.

He had been the senior of two partners in a small accountancy firm for ten years, and then had had an offer of amalgamation from a multinational accountancy business. This offer would be financially beneficial, give more long-term security, and provide a wider range of professional skills for the clients. On the debit side, he would lose the independence of being his own boss and the satisfaction that brings. In the end he decided to accept the offer, but his wife was totally opposed to it and thought it would not be for the best; his secretary also held this view. During the year following the integration, he had gradually become aware of frictions between the executive staff. His clients did not like the less personalized service, while he himself felt rather dissatisfied. He could not share these feelings with his wife or his secretary because they had been adamantly against the change.

After two visits, during which he quietly expressed much frustration and anger, his depression lifted and his sexual libido returned. However, the problem recurred a few months later when his firm discovered they had overpaid him and his ex-partner by a large sum of money, which had to be repaid. In order to do this quickly he had to increase the mortgage on his house, which had been transferred to his wife's name some years before; therefore her agreement was essential. In anger she said, 'You haven't got a house!'

This man developed some insight into how his depression and anger made life less enjoyable, and had aroused mixed feelings towards his wife. He thought that he might be able to deal with these feelings more appropriately, but knew he found it difficult to fight his battles openly. Therefore, he thought he would 'withdraw' from the managerial role he held within the firm. The interpretation of the behaviour was shared between the doctor and the patient with the laughter of understanding. Having developed some insight into the cause of his sexual problem, he may be able to deal with his conflicting emotions more realistically.

RELATIONSHIP PROBLEMS

The most common cause of loss of libido is everyday difficulty within a relationship. Often the couple is unaware that their sexual behaviour is mirroring their unconscious hostile feelings in the same way as it might their loving ones. Ambivalence to the partner may be wrapped up in protestations of peace and harmony, such as, 'We hardly ever quarrel. We've only had one or two rows in the whole of our married life. I love my husband (wife) very much, but . . .' There usually follows many wishes that the spouse were different.

An incredible amount of resentment can come from an overtly loving woman, who is puzzled by her loss of interest in sex. A life event, such as living together, marriage, or childbirth may have accentuated the relationship problems and triggered the symptom. Similar resentments may be heard from men who declare that they have a very happy marriage: 'She never seems to have time for me now that we have two children. Of course, she does still manage to go to her flower club and visit her sister most days. She chats with her brainy friends and I feel that I'm not good enough for her and I often feel shut out.'

The anger is expressed by sexual withdrawal. These mixed feelings present a dilemma both to the patient and to the doctor. The pretence of uncontaminated love acts as a defence against angry feelings. This defence has to be lowered if the battle between the sheets is to be recognized. It is said that women will not and men cannot – sexual withdrawal from the partner is a very potent weapon. The defence of love and happiness protects the psyche from the pain of recognizing the bad feelings and the despair which might put the relationship in serious jeopardy. Thus the hostility is unconscious and symbolized by the sexual problem.

A dark, attractive microbiology student aged 29 was referred to the family planning clinic with the symptom of loss of libido and difficulty in reaching orgasm of about six months. Intelligent and articulate, she could not understand why she felt so sexually withdrawn from her husband, who is 'such a nice guy'. They had been married for ten years. He was 39 and a PhD student in a scientific subject. They both came from traditional Middle East families, and had come to England because of political troubles. It had become obvious they would never return.

During the consultation, she first told of what a marvellous man she had married and how much they loved each other. Then little criticisms began to emerge. Her resentment had increased recently because a couple, who were friends of her husband's extended family, came to live with them while staying in England for a major surgical operation. She did not know them previously, and did not like them at all. They were not clean and tidy enough in the house, and she did not like cleaning up after them and providing a taxi service to the hospital, and so on. She felt her husband should have been much more active in looking after them. Gradually, the extent of her angry feelings towards her husband became clear. Ever since they had married ten years ago he had been more interested in abstract political ideas than in completing his thesis and getting a job. He did not need to earn money because his family was wealthy. She was employed by a hospital department and about to achieve her degree. She also told of her sadness about separation from her parents, whereas she was angry with her father-in-law, who had written a very critical letter to them.

This patient made various practical excuses to discontinue the consultation with the doctor, probably because she did not wish to share her exposed anger against her husband with the doctor, which might be threatening to her marriage. She could not face the fact that there was a major marital disharmony lying behind her loss of libido.

A defence against dependence

A GP referred a 25-year-old girl to the psychosexual clinic complaining of lack of lubrication during inter-course and having to use K-Y jelly as a substitute. She was a heavily built, rather tomboyish girl in jeans who was cheerful and at ease with the doctor. She described the symptom, adding she could reach orgasm, but needed to use the jelly for the last few months, whereas previously she was easily aroused and lubricated well. Her medical record card showed she was a bank cashier and her boyfriend was a welder. This social difference gave the doctor a possible clue to the difficulty, and he asked about the idea of marriage. The patient quickly explained that she did not want to marry for at least two years because she had a nice bungalow of her own, whereas her boyfriend still lived with his mother. She took in lodgers to help pay the mortgage, but her boy-friend wanted her to get rid of them; then he would come and live with her. They definitely could not afford to do that because he had such a low wage, and, she added, 'I enjoy having the lodgers anyway.'

Her boyfriend also resented the fact that she belonged

to the Territorial Army, for which not only was she paid but which was a source of companionship and enjoyment for her. Clearly, the conflict between them was reducing her libido, giving the need for artificial lubrication. Once she was physically involved she surrendered to the pleasure and reached orgasm. The doctor pointed out her independence and her capability in running her own life, and how, in contrast, she saw her partner as being a poor wage-earner, with less social ability and a need to have her exclusively to himself. She said disparagingly that his only other interest was Friday night out in the pub 'with the boys'.

If, with the doctor's help, this patient develops insight, the relationship may founder; the sexual difficulty she is experiencing is the symptom of a fairly profound conflict. This girl needed to choose a partner who was not her equal educationally or in earning capacity, but on the other hand despised his inadequacies and was unable to allow herself to be dependent upon him. She had to be the boss, which was a defence against her fear of any weakness or dependency within herself.

ANGER BEHIND THE NEED TO PLEASE

A man's apparent need to please the woman can hide a great deal of hostility. In constantly employing a placatory role, he is unaware of the anger this engenders within himself. The manifestation of this anger may be loss of libido, premature ejaculation, or even impotence.

A married couple attended the doctor together. It soon became obvious that the husband was there only because his wife wished him to be, and he was not motivated at that time to seek help for himself. She blamed their unsatisfactory sex life for the unhappiness within the marriage. She said that intercourse was very infrequent, and made many derogatory remarks about his lack of skill as a lover: 'He always seems to touch me in the wrong places.'

The man had been a virgin when they married, whereas she had previously been married and divorced. In contrast to how it was in bed, she said he would do many things which she liked, such as always remembering her birthday and their anniversary, and sending cards and flowers. He was also a good vegetable gardener and grew beautiful, fresh vegetables for her to cook with. She expressed appreciation that he was thoughtful in planning surprise visits to a theatre or concert, and so in some ways knew she was lucky – but he did not know how to make love, and he never showed any passion. Her husband agreed with his wife during the consultation, and made no protest at her criticisms. The doctor decided to see them individually. (The therapy of the wife will not be described here.)

When seen alone, the husband was surprised at the doctor's comment about his passive and placatory attitude in the previous encounter, but he gradually began to express many resentments against his wife's dominance, which often assumed a kind of parental role and brooked no argument. He placated her rather than have a stand-up fight. To compensate for his angry feelings he would be especially nice to her, giving the impression of being a loving and considerate husband, providing treats and flowers. Overtly he did everything to please her, but his resentment made him a slavish, ineffectual lover who could not take charge of the situation and therefore lacked spontaneity and passion. Until the hostility behind the façade of devotion could be understood by the man, the need to please would be seen as a virtue rather than as a defence against real feelings.

This man was repeating behaviour patterns learned in childhood and adolescence from having been brought up in an all-female environment. His father left home when he was ten years old, and with his mother and two younger sisters he went to live with their grandmother. He felt a great responsibility in being the only man of the household, and grew up a very sensible son and older brother, and controlled his less acceptable feelings. His more childlike impulses and spontaneity were suppressed, and with them his sexual passion.

MOURNING

Grief is a potent inhibitor of sexual feelings, especially when the feelings of sadness are complicated by guilt, or even relief, over a death. Mourning does not occur only for a loved person, but also for other kinds of loss, such as fertility, youth, or after a hysterectomy.

The patient had a total hysterectomy for menorrhagia and a colpo suspension for stress incontinence three years ago. The reason for the present referral was an eight-week history of lack of interest in sexual activity. Previously it had been rewarding, and had been fully restored after the gynaecological operations, which had improved her life enormously, after being troubled by menstrual symptoms for years. During the consultation the patient almost immediately began to talk about the death of her mother, with whom she had had an unsatisfactory relationship. When her mother had become ill, she would not come and live with her daughter, although she could not manage on her own. Her mother had requested specific funeral arrangements, but these could not be carried out because the local parson was on holiday. The patient had an undue feeling of guilt about this, and mourning for her mother became full of confused feelings and 'if only's'.

Her one uncritical friend and comfort had always been her dog, who had died soon after her mother. In telling of this event, although it happened almost a year ago, she had tears in her eyes. She desperately wanted another dog, but her husband felt they should not have any more because of the difficulty of its care when taking holidays. She knew this was rational and sensible, but could not come to terms with this decision. His attitudes were more pragmatic than hers, and she felt he could not share the pain of her loss – so the sexual barriers were built between them. With some insight into her feelings, she began to feel better and enjoy her sexual life again.

In this case it is interesting to note that the moment of greatest emotion was when the patient was talking about the loss of her dog, rather than her mother's death as might have been expected.

These feelings were related to the present situation with her husband. He did not understand her loss, her sense of being alone, or her 'irrational' need for another dog. It is not surprising that her unrecognized anger with her husband for his inability to understand her grief expressed itself by sexual withdrawal.

A 32-year-old woman was referred by her family planning clinic doctor for loss of libido of about one year. The referral letter had questioned whether the termination of a pregnancy could have been the aetiological factor. The patient, who was a professional press photographer, was a little sad in demeanour and lacking in vivacity, but very articulate. She too wondered if the termination was relevant to her sexual disinterest. She was on the brink of tears as she began to present the problem to the doctor, but soon gained control and was able to discuss very rationally her decision not to continue wih her pregnancy, of which she became aware while taking photographs in the war-stricken area of Ethiopia. She returned to Zimbabwe, where she and her boyfriend, a geologist, had been living and working for a time. After discussing it with him, she flew to England for the operation. She felt at the time it was the right decision because the relationship had been brief, and she did not feel ready to bring up a baby in view of her professional lifestyle.

The sexual relationship with her boyfriend had been mutually rewarding, but now she never felt she wanted to have intercourse, and never enjoyed it fully when she did. She was puzzled why this was, because the relationship in all other ways seemed to be fine. They had now moved back to England, were both employed and shared a house together. Both had had previous long-term relationships, but this one was for her the most satisfactory, except for her poor sexual libido.

She went on to tell the doctor more about her life and work and how she had been banned from Zimbabwe because of political problems over some of her work. The ban was very quickly lifted, but nevertheless it was a great shock at the time. It probably was a factor in the decision to return to England about seven months ago. The doctor pointed out how barriers seem to have been put up around her, and she said, 'I don't even seem to be able to talk to my friends as I used to do. There seems no point.'

At this moment the atmosphere was such that the doctor said, 'It sounds as though you feel that you've been kicked in the stomach.' Then the tears fell as she said, 'Well, you see, my mother died. I came home from Africa three months before she died, but she had never told me how ill she was. She was a really super and interesting person, and often used to write to me while I was away. She wouldn't have wanted me to have left my work and come home, which is probably why she didn't tell us that she had cancer. I can't talk about it to anyone because my sister has had post-natal depression recently, and my father manages very well, but I don't want to upset him.' The tears were settling, so the doctor could interpret the unfinished business of mourning, which had been delayed by the involvement in the decision about the pregnancy and its termination. The pain of her mother's death was being relived by her return to England, because previously whenever she had come home her mother had been there, and she had enjoyed her affection and company.

Putting this young woman in touch with her unfinished grieving may help her to understand her loss of libido, and to be able to complete the mourning process.

Again, this case illustrates the need for the doctor to follow the patient beyond what may appear to be an adequate explanation for the loss of libido, in this case the termination, to whatever point of deep emotional pain the patient may discover. Only then will healing be able to begin.

It is not, however, always possible to separate out the exact emotional cause of sexual withdrawal. Sometimes the bereaved person is unable to open out to the intensity of sexual feeling for fear of being open to the full force of the grief. In other cases there may be several layers of feeling related to different circumstances that need to be worked through in the presence of a listening doctor.

POST-NATAL DISTURBANCE

Loss of libido after a baby may result from a change of feeling about the self, due to the experience of pregnancy and childbirth. For instance, the woman may feel profoundly damaged, or the man may feel unable to cope with the feelings of what he may have caused his spouse to endure. The childbirth experience is certainly not always totally happy and joyful. Many women hate the loss of their independence and the exposure of feelings during childbirth, and some are haunted by the memory of fear and pain. Relationship problems may occur after the arrival of a baby because of the emotional adjustments needed in the change from being a couple to being parents. A jealous, disturbed husband revealed his feelings by pinning a 'No Visitors' sign on his wife's ward door in the hospital. He could not stand her being congratulated and given flowers, nor the thought of his rival the baby, at the foot of the bed. In the post-partum days, echoes of the woman's own childhood sadness may impair her sexual pleasure, because becoming a mother makes her relive these feelings. The subject of problems related to childbirth is explored further in Chapter 10,

SELF-PUNISHMENT OR CONTROL

There may be unconscious inhibition of sexuality by a need to atone for life's events, such as the termination of pregnancy or earlier promiscuity, or a control exerted for fear of being like a parent whose sexual life led to family distress in the past. Cervical dysplasia and malignant disease are known to be related to early adolescent sexual intercourse, multiple partners, and also a male factor. Knowledge of the risk factors may have a profound emotional effect on patients and their partners who have this pathology. Remembrance of previous sexuality may inhibit the woman from sexual libido, and the partners of women who develop genital disease may also withdraw from them because of guilt or distress.

> Jennie, an attractive, intelligent girl in her late 20s consulted her doctor about her complete loss of libido. She had had cervical dysplasia and laser treatment 18 months before. She lived with her boyfriend, with whom the relationship seemed settled, rewarding, and satisfac-

tory, but she was completely disinterested in sex. She and the doctor explored her attitude to the relationship and her life in general, but there did not appear to be anything outstandingly wrong, except for the absence of sexual libido. In her late adolescence she had had a very rebellious and promiscuous phase; the rebellion seemed to be against her mother, and she said, 'My mother is always shouting,' and she felt her sister had always been preferred by her mother.

After three visits, during which doctor and patient puzzled together, she volunteered that she just seemed to feel fear when she thought of having sexual intercourse. At this point it was possible to interpret to her the disgust she felt about the promiscuous stage of her life and her own disapproval of her passionate but superficial sexuality, and her guilt about the previous malignant disease of the cervix. Jennie was able to discuss her ambivalent feelings when it came to the point of having intercourse. She really wanted to enjoy it, and yet she shut down these feelings of enjoyment, retreated from it, and switched off at the last moment.

Having shared with the doctor her feelings of disapproval of herself, and also her fear of the recurrence of the dysplasia, her libido began to recover and gradually her sexual pleasure returned.

The need for self-punishment after what is felt to have been unacceptable behaviour has been called 'The wrath of the gods syndrome'. Doctors working in the field of colcoscopy of urogenital medicine need to be alert to the effect that such investigations and treatment may have on sexual relationships.

THE THERAPEUTIC ENCOUNTER

To treat this symptom, whatever its aetiology, it is necessary for the doctor in the neutral and trusted atmosphere of the consultation to help the patient to share and accept painful truths that previously have been unconscious. The true emotions can then often be accepted, with a tribute to their existence. Resentments in relationships can be dealt with in a more appropriate manner than by sexual withdrawal; a power struggle is better settled with an overt row than covert hostility. The doctor can point out the part the patient is playing in the problem, and help him/her to express anger and fear so that there is some option for change, with a restoration of sexual libido and more effective communication with the partner. The common aetiological factor in so many cases of loss of libido is unconscious anger, which can be directed at life, at the self, the partner, or other significant figures in that person's life, such as a parent. The task of the doctor is to help the patient to lower the defences enough to make these feelings conscious, more appropriately directed, and more acceptable.

10

Pregnancy, childbirth and female sexuality

Alexandra Tobart

SUMMARY

- Being a woman
- The meaning of being a wife
- Sexual difficulties during pregnancy
- Childbirth
- Feelings about being a mother
- The baby as a reminder

In order to understand the sexual difficulties which arise during pregnancy and in the post-natal period, it is helpful to consider the development of sexual maturity in general; the nature of its well-being, and the impediments to its achievement.

The expression of sexual feelings depends upon the resolution of a conflict which arises inevitably between opposing emotional forces. On the one hand there is sexual desire and need, and the yearning to love and to be loved; on the other there is the repressive power of fear and anger: fear of too great an intensity of

Source: *Midwife, Health Visitor and Community Nurse*, Vol. 26, Nos 7 and 8, pp. 177–80, 1990

feeling and thence of loss of control; fear of vulnerability and helplessness, of physical and emotional exposure; fear of loss of dignity and of mess. Anger is usually related to the experience or observation of relationships that appeared to cause pain rather than contentment. The various aspects of this conflict and the balance between them have their foundation in the individual's unique history. Often, hopefully most often, the conflict is resolved by a victory of the positive forces, but even when a satisfactory balance has been achieved, there will be events and circumstances during life that will re-awaken echoes from the past, which may again disturb the balance.

A child is vulnerable and largely helpless. If that condition is respected and protected, from such care will grow a healthy tolerance of an adult's weakness and that of others, and a realization that strength and weakness are not alternatives but can exist in harmonious togetherness. It is interesting that in many cases the fear of vulnerability and helplessness is found to be an important factor when sexual difficulties arise during pregnancy and in the post-natal period.

BEING A WOMAN

Most women find contentment and satisfaction in their femininity and enjoy their relationships with each other and with men. The times of difficulty and struggle are usually met with courage and determination. There are some unhappy women, however, for whom all feminine functions are burdensome, from menarche to menopause. Painful menstruation, symptomful pregnancy, difficult births, problems of child-bearing all form a sad progression towards a suffering middle age. Times of physiological transition become crises of emotional instability. Sadly, the absence of happy sex is often another feature in this picture of troubled femininity.

Frigidity in all its many manifestations, temporarily or persistently may take its place in the symptom complex of troubled femininity. In terms which do not explore, but at the same time do not deny or contradict, the analytical understanding of early childhood development, femininity may be likened to an heirloom which requires to be handed on from mother to daughter in an unconscious, intangible ceremonial. Many patients describe how mother died or departed; or lived unloving, unloved, or unfaithful;

or how she refused to come to her daughter's wedding or to help with the baby.

Thus there is an interruption of the psychological ceremonial and a break in the continuity. In differing ways and for differing reasons the heirloom of femininity was not offered or not acceptable, and the daughter is left bereft and unable to function in wholeness. One deeply troubled woman, who had been describing her demanding, unsupporting mother, was asked about her grandmother. She said, despairingly, 'Like my mother, only worse.'

THE MEANING OF BEING A WIFE

Pregnancy, childbirth, and the post-natal period sometimes bring into the open feelings about what it is to be a wife which were not apparent in the exciting days of courtship and the time of marriage without children. The achievements of women in their struggle to move forward from the position which generations before them had to tolerate have led to untold benefits, but inevitably there have been problems too. No longer are women compelled by their material dependence, re-enforced by their inability to control their fertility, to live in obedience, sometimes in subjection, to their lord and master.

Many couples have achieved a comfortable balance in which each makes an individual and appropriate contribution to the well-being of the family. For some, however, marriage becomes a competition. Particularly when a wife has achieved material and social status and the accompanying self-reliance, the daily life of a woman running a home and looking after her husband and children, thoroughly enjoyed by many women, may feel like a relegation to a backwater of life. Sexuality, which could provide joyful, shared togetherness, becomes a battleground.

Mrs A had lived with her future husband for several years, during which time both had thoroughly enjoyed their careers and also their many shared activities. Their sexual life was happy and satisfactory for both. They then decided they wanted a child, and that they would marry when Mrs A became pregnant. After their son was born, Mrs A became increasingly bad-tempered. She complained she was trapped, while her husband, a hard-working office manager, had all the fun. When he came home she petulantly provided a no-trouble meal, and complained that he would not talk to her. Almost always she refused his sexual advances. In relation to this, and much else, her oft-repeated phrase was, 'I don't want it.'

Pregnancy, and the months of adapting to the changes which the need to care for a child will bring about, challenge all the feelings a woman has about herself as a woman, a wife, and a mother. The father of the child has of course a crucial role to play by giving his support and demonstrating his willingness to share the tasks with loving enthusiasm.

Perhaps we do not give enough thought to the desperate loneliness of a woman bearing a child no man wants. Many women, and even young girls, face such a situation with great courage, but it is one where family, friends, and professional helpers have a vital role to play.

SEXUAL DIFFICULTIES DURING PREGNANCY

During pregnancy some women may refuse intercourse for many months, often justifying this attitude by insisting the baby might be damaged. It is probable that this fear is based not on logic but upon an identification with the small, weak being inside that cannot defend itself and must be protected.

Most pregnant women feel intensely protective towards the baby inside but sometimes there is instead a bitter antagonism. A patient seen recently, who had a severely obsessional personality focused upon the fear that whatever came from within her was bad, found her pregnant body disgusting, and later had great difficulty believing that her healthy baby was good and clean. For many months every nappy change remained a crisis, and her son was more than a year old before she felt deeply loving towards him. She has not so far resumed her sexual life.

CHILDBIRTH

For some women, the experience of childbirth is accompanied by almost unbearable feelings of physical and emotional exposure, as well as loss of control and dignity. Their fear of 'letting go' may be evident in the progress, or lack of progress, of labour. They may be seen as irritable and irritating patients, and test the sensitivity of the most kindly nurses and doctors, who may later be described in the most derogatory terms. The husband, particularly when sexual intercourse is attempted, later may provide a further focus for this defensive anger.

Dyspareunia

Sometimes the absence of sexual responsiveness is justified by a complaint of pain or soreness. On examination there may be evidence of an unsatisfactory repair of a tear or an episiotomy, which requires attention. Often, however, nothing abnormal is found, but the patient's sense of having been damaged remains. It is clearly important to respond with respect and concern, and to help the patient to find and to accept her physical health.

In dealing with sexual difficulties after childbirth, the patient often leads the discussion to the details of labour and birth. The impression emerges that this potentially joyful event was perceived as a kind of rape. Indeed, such very different experiences are often expressed in strikingly similar terms, the outstanding feature being the sense of angry helplessness, which remains with the woman long and painfully, and continues to impede happy sexuality. During treatment, a history of earlier traumatic experiences sometimes emerges and demands attention.

Mrs B, a woman of 32, had postponed pregnancy for 10 years because she was terrified of childbirth. Finally, her own and her husband's wish for a child had helped her to find courage. She found the birth a horrendous experience, and lost all sexual feeling thereafter. Almost immediately she led the discussion to the memory of being raped not long before her marriage. Without prompting she related the details of that terrifying event several times. Gradually she realized that her feelings about childbirth bore a remarkable similarity to the earlier attack. During treatment this insight helped her to separate the two events, so that the earlier no longer overshadowed the later. Before long she found a new joy in her son, and in her sexual relationship with her husband.

FEELINGS ABOUT BEING A MOTHER

The demands made by a new baby draw upon all the mother's emotional reserves. Hopefully these reserves have been laid down in childhood, re-stocked from fulfilling relationships throughout life, and consistently replenished in marriage by a loving husband whose affection she is able to accept and to absorb. Sadly, such experiences have not been a part of life for many women, who have to struggle unsupported, sometimes unloved, to fulfil the needs of their child. To give when too little has been received, in the past and present, is a daunting challenge, courageously faced by many women, but sometimes impossible to meet.

Heather was 26, plump, and pretty. She had been married for seven years, and had two daughters aged four years and 18 months. She came for help because since the birth of her second child she had lost all interest in sex, feeling miserable, and realizing that her marriage, which had before been warm and happy, both sexually and generally, was deteriorating. She was also worried because she was readily loving to the baby, but short-tempered with her older child.

During her second pregnancy, Heather's parents had separated. Logically, she thought this was a good thing because they had fought all their lives, but to her surprise she found herself very upset and her parents constantly on her mind both in the present and in memories of her childhood. She described her father as a drinker and a liar, and her mother as a nagger. Many incidents emerged of her mother's coldness and lack of sensitivity to the feelings of her family. Neither parent offered physical affection. Heather was the eldest of three girls, and much had been expected of her regarding sensible adult behaviour; she felt very responsible for her sisters. She depicted with modest pride the contrast both materially and emotionally between her squalid childhood home and the home which she and her husband had created. She was terrified now of spoiling it by her coldness to her husband and her irritability with her elder daughter. She was particularly shocked when she heard herself saying to her husband, 'Get off, it's my body, not yours,' in the same tone she had heard her mother use when as a child she pulled the blankets over her head so as not to hear her parents quarrelling.

Heather came to see that although her childhood had provided a poor foundation for her adult femininity, her own personality had been sound enough to overcome these handicaps – until the vulnerable time of her second pregnancy and her parents' separation had disturbed the balance. She also believed she was treating her elder daughter as she felt she had been treated herself, by denying her the opportunity of being a child.

A happy sexual life is without doubt a most potent source of emotional support at a time when so much giving is required. Often the early weeks and months of motherhood are an exhausting process of work and worry, when sexual intercourse is seen as just another demand when all the mother wants to do is to sleep.

A most significant source of support in the post-natal period is the mother's mother. The daughter is fortunate indeed if her own mother has provided a model of healthy feminity, and is available to offer emotional and practical help. This has the effect of supporting her daughter's confidence, and does not induce a sense of inferiority, rivalry or guilt.

Post-natal loss of libido is a very common condition which threatens the stability of a marriage and thence the well-being of the family as a whole. In many cases it becomes clear that the sexual difficulty exists as a remnant of an earlier post-natal depression, or as a concomitant of one which has settled into an ongoing chronic state. The mother is tired and increasingly bad-tempered. A lack of energy and enthusiasm pervades her daily life, and makes all that has to be done effortful and joyless. Her husband is puzzled and often resentful, complaining that nothing he does pleases his wife. His sexual approaches are not seen as loving, but as demanding.

Those whose help is sought – GPs, midwives, health visitors, or doctors working in psychosexual medicine – may find it difficult to see a way out of the overwhelming gloom and despondency. Antidepressant medication may be prescribed and may be of temporary benefit, but will hardly help the sufferer come to grips with the heart of the problem. If the woman can be helped to form a sound treatment relationship with her chosen helper, it is likely that insight and understanding will grow and will form the basis of change. Most commonly, the story which emerges centres around the patient's own childhood experience – the love and security which was or was not offered, and the traumas which overshadowed it.

THE BABY AS A REMINDER

For some women, their own baby on an unconscious level represents a younger sibling who aroused feelings which could not be expressed or resolved. It is almost inevitable that an older child should feel jealousy and anger, often of great intensity, towards a new baby. It is not easy for parents to love and support a child through such feelings, which must then be repressed and covered by 'good' feelings. Sometimes depression results, but commonly there is the development of a personality that is self-disciplined, hard-working and orderly, and which functions fully and effectively. Vulnerability lies in situations which provoke dependence and guilt.

Many years later, the arrival of her own baby may re-awaken repressed feelings and result in all or part of a post-partum symptom complex of depression, withdrawal from affection, anger towards the child, and intense anxiety. During treatment it is likely to be difficult for the patient to accept that such feelings lie deep within her, but once she can do so, a new freedom will be reached.

> Clare was a young teacher who was seen when her first baby, Emma, was eight months old. She had been clinically depressed almost immediately after Emma's birth, and had been treated with antidepressants. She had improved and was now looking after her baby very well, but she remained tense, anxious, and tearful, and had lost all her previously healthy sexual feelings. Above all, she was deeply distressed by the feelings of resentment and occasional near violence which she had experienced towards Emma. 'That isn't me,' she declared.
>
> Clare had taught until she was seven months' pregnant. Emma was a much-wanted child. Her husband was also a teacher, who proved to be unfailingly loving although much absorbed in his own work. She spoke

with deep affection of her own mother and of her happy childhood. She had one sister, three years younger, who had been a sickly, crying baby. Clare had a few memories of her early childhood, but often said she was thought of as being a very good child. It proved necessary to work slowly to help Clare to accept her own aggressive feelings, which had appeared so out of place in her kindly childhood home and too frightening in their intensity to be expressed towards her sister.

There are other echoes from the past which impede adult happiness. One patient who presented with post-natal depression and total loss of sexual interest had been hospitalized for many months in early childhood because of severe orthopaedic deformity. She had grown up to be a mature and confident adult, but this achievement was shattered when her second child was found to have the same deformity. During treatment she relived all the feelings of helplessness, anger, and despair which had been so overwhelming in her early life.

It is well known that child abuse is most damaging to later emotional and sexual development. The effects of such damage are likely to be most severe during pregnancy and in the post-natal period.

Bereavement which occurs close to pregnancy is particularly hard to overcome. To feel the sadness of death and the gladness of birth imposes a severe emotional challenge which often needs much support and help, without which ongoing depression may result.

Well-being depends upon a sound balance between that which is taken in and that which is given out. This applies to many areas of life: the physical, in terms of food and energy; the financial in terms of the bank account; and very clearly to the emotional aspects of being.

If parents are able to absorb love and sexual fulfilment from each other there will almost certainly be a beneficial effect upon the quality of their relationship with their children. Nevertheless, it is almost certainly true that there are many mothers and fathers whose inner resources are sufficiently healthy to meet the challenge of parenting without the added support of a satisfying sexual life. The increasing divorce rate among the parents of young children demands concerned understanding of its causes and its effects.

Whatever conclusions are reached, any help which can be made available to overcome sexual difficulties will be of long-term benefit. That is our role. It would be hard to find a more challenging and rewarding area of preventive medicine.

11

On female sexuality

Tom Main

SUMMARY

- Images of motherhood
- The missing man
- Finding the genitals
- Loving as well as hating
- Defences
- Maturational hurdles
- Dealing with guilt and anxiety
- Puberty
- Adult problems

As with most features of adulthood, if we are to understand final adult female sexuality we need to know what has gone on before. Yet questions such as – How does it begin? What are the early physical and mental developments and how do they mutually influence each other during growth? – are too big for this chapter. Even one part of the subject, such as developments at puberty

Source: *The Journal of Family Planning Doctors* (now *British Journal of Family Planning*) (1977), **2**(4), 61 and 64–6. ©.

(of body and mind and the growth of sexual fantasies about boys and breasts and periods, of idealizing being in love and mate-seeking) is formidable; while disorders of pubertal development (shyness, dysmenorrhoea, disgust and depression, guilt about and fears of sexual excitement, resentment of hair, and breasts and periods and boys, overeating and anorexia) is worthy of separate consideration. If it is also remembered that each maturational feat not only of puberty but of courtship, marriage, consummation, of pregnancy, labour, lactation, and of mothering had its precursors from infancy onwards it will be clear the most to be aimed at in any short statement is the discussion of one single line of feminine development, thus to lift it out of context and to pay the inevitable price of distorted emphasis. I propose therefore to discuss a little and yet a lot – some effects on adult sexual functioning of the girl's early relation to the mother.

IMAGES OF MOTHERHOOD

The very word 'mother' is often sentimentalized because it can so easily evoke in everyone images of tender care, devotion and sweetness. Such images pay tribute to the states of bliss, of which all infants must have a minimum if they are to survive, and to the infant's total unguarded helpless adoration of the mother at such times. This serene madonna image therefore enshrines a truth about early human experience, but sadly only a one-sided truth.

There is also the other side of the mother/child relationship, the infantile rages and hatred and terrors which every mother regularly inspires in her child because of the inevitable frustrations she is experienced as imposing. Such experiences temporarily blot out the love of the madonna-mother and lead the infant to different, equally distorted, images. It now knows it has an evil monstrous mother who hates and tortures and starves and gloats at the terror of helpless babies.

The madonna and the witch; each is a derivative image of the mother as she is variously felt to be; and each is extreme, simply because in early life states of love and hatred are themselves extreme. With children there are no half-measures. Mummy is not fairly good; she is the most lovely mummy in the whole world and she is the best cook and the prettiest and we love her for ever and ever and ever. And now she is the most horrible mummy anybody ever had and we hate her and will only be happy after she's dead and will never, never forgive her. Never, never, never.

THE MISSING MAN

We can easily note that these two extreme images – which are indeed the child's reality – contain another interesting blindness. The mother, be she madonna or witch, is simply a woman whose only interest in life is loving or hating the child. But as in the pre-Renaissance pictures of madonna and child there is a missing figure; there is no man. These primitive mothers of the infant, marvellous or evil, have no sexual partner. This is the result of the belief of the infant that it is the centre of the world and that the mother – good or bad – belongs only to him and that her sole motive is to arrange things perfectly or abominably for him. He is her one and only and it is inconceivable that she could have any other interest. Father too is only a father; that is his job; and he too belongs only to the child and functions only for him. The fact that the woman is primarily a wife not a mother and the man primarily a husband not a father, and that they belong primarily to each other with the child a mere by-blow of their relationship is not known to the infant. Mummy is a mummy and daddy is a daddy; and that's that. And that's all.

Later, the growing evidence that his parents can and do relate to each other more than they relate to him is outrageous and humiliating. This idea rocks the whole comfortable world of the infant and is therefore hotly resisted. The first arrangement, with the infant the supreme centre of the universe and the others as his satellite possessions is something to fight for. The growing child now rages at and resents any parental pairing which excludes him. His rageful refusal to contemplate exclusion gets noisy testimony at bedtime in many homes with children of one to three. Sleeplessness, the wish to be in mummy's bed, requests for a drink of water, and so on are common results of this struggle against the two.

FINDING THE GENITALS

But another development coincides more or less with this onset of rage and jealousy at the idea that the parents are owned by each other and that the child is small-fry. By the age of one most normal children have found their own genitals and as the months pass they can rely on them to give pleasure as well as comfort in times of trouble. This makes the situation better in the sense that the child no longer depends only on the mother for comfort, and yet it also makes it worse. The growing child eventually suspects not only that each parent can give himself the same genital pleasure, but eventually worse still that they do blissful and rude and exciting things to each other when they are together without him. They not only give each other lovely drinks and food and play rude games with each other's bottoms and 'poo-poo' and 'wee-wee', but also have lovely fun with each other's genitals.

As he grows and his interest in genitals grows many signs will confirm his highly imaginative suspicions about their other secrets, including their capacity to make babies, and now the fat is truly in the fire. His majesty, the centre of the world, loyal and needy, is deserted and betrayed by those very people he worshipped and trusted and depended on. Degraded to unthinkable satellite status, he is left at the mercy of new murderous rages at the newly perceived triangular situation, with violent jealousies about the excitingly rude orgies he imagines his parents enjoy and from which he – the only one who matters – is cruelly excluded. This situation is the more enraging and painful because the toddler, still helplessly dependent on his parents, has now grown an active sexual curiosity which is inevitably unsatisfied and unsatisfiable. Their selfishness is criminal. The father can give mother a baby – why should he prefer her? In simple justice why cannot he give one to his daughter, the really important person?

The father's callous crime is compounded by the faithless mother – unbelievably selfish she refuses to yield to the child the wicked and lovely and nameless pleasures she gets from the father. She will not even share it. Nor will the father. These wicked parents shut their lovely child out of their disgraceful conspiracy of mysterious ecstasies. In his loneliest rages the child hates them and develops envious fantasies in which he fashions revenges with his own genitals and bottom to destroy their pleasures and filthy up their joys. And serve them right.

LOVING AS WELL AS HATING

From this basic situation, inevitable because of the developments of love and hate and egocentricity and bodily functions and growing sexual interest, many developments may flow. There follow a few extreme possibilities.

First – and we must remember this – the child also loves his/her parents, and thus may get frightened of his/her rages and destructive thoughts and seek to control these. The girl child may develop a concerned over-protectiveness towards her mother, may worry about her happiness, feel responsible if daddy gets angry at mummy and may feel wicked at having any ambitions of her own about daddy. Overly good and devoted, the girl may worry about how mummy will cope if the girl is not there to protect her from catastrophes. Now, clinging and fearful of parting from mummy, the girl is set for phobias about school, and about the crime of growing up and away into sexuality of her own. She may be set never to be free, always to look after and consult mummy, to live always near perhaps never to leave her parental home and never to enjoy her own body except with anxiety and guilt about trespassing into mummy's territory.

Second, the girl may be so ambivalent about her mother, especially if the maternal care is indifferent, that her love is regularly swamped by hatred so that she comes to fear and expect just retaliation for her sexual jealousies and rages. She may now see in her mother's discipline, not a forgivable mummy, but simply evidence that her mother hates her in turn and especially her femininity, her sexual curiosities and her early maternal ambitions. The way is now open for later terrors at sexual growth because it is felt to be anti-mother, rivalrous, forbidden and punishable.

A third possibility is that the toddler's love for her mother may be so steady, in spite of her hatred, that it can mitigate her destructive energy. In place of envy there grows admiration of the mother for having such marvellous and beautiful bodily powers and sexuality, and such cleverness at attracting daddy and making babies, together with a wish to be like her, loving and lovable. Because of this love she may come, by projection, to believe that her mother in turn is equally friendly towards her own feminine ambitions and will support this as she grows up. Such a girl acquires an early blessing within herself and confidently welcomes her later feminine developments with the same pride as she had in her mother's achievements.

A fourth possibility is that, in rage at a mother who prefers doing rude and filthy sexy things with a man to caring for sad and lonely little girls, the infant may come to see her mother as a faithless prostitute. This hating picture of the mother who, I remind you, is also loved, is usually so unbearable that desperate mental defences against it are set up.

DEFENCES

The most common is a regressive step to the earlier idealized image – the madonna, sweet, immaculate and clean, a two-body figure only, without the man of the painful eternal triangle. This mother loves only babies and never enjoys rude behaviour with daddy. It is only he who is excited by rude and cruel sexy things – mummy only shuts her eyes and puts up with his dirty behaviour. It gives her no pleasure – in fact it hurts her and when she does it, it is only to appease a brute. When she conceived the girl she was not thinking of enjoyment with the man – only about the little baby girl to come. This fantasy of mother, sweet, suffering and anti-sex is a fairly common model for girls. Indeed this model may govern her later life – whereby she too suffers the dirty appetites of men, sex and childbirth in the noble sacrifice of mothering. Such women are devoted to their children and to mothering, but give their husbands no status and no joys. One variety of this development is the Polly Garter woman, promiscuous but always getting pregnant, occupied essentially with baby-making and despising men and sexuality.

These are four extreme illustrative possibilities of development. These extreme pictures are not very common but minor elements of all four are to be found frequently. Moreover all four can alternate – depending on the current life situation of the image-maker. Such developments are however usually fateful for the girl's final development as a woman. This is because by the age of six most of this imagery has become unconscious and is therefore relatively unmodifiable. A bias of the girl about her mother and about her own femininity is thus laid down early in life, and the ways she will view and understand later experiences are heavily affected by this bias. This bias will dog all of her feminine developments including her relations with men and she will escape from it only by rare good luck in such matters as her choice of husband.

There is of course great variety of bias, of kind and intensity, but in general it is the way a little girl surmounts her mother's essential infidelity which leads her either to pride and pleasure or to imagined reproaches and disapprovals and sufferings by her mother as she grows her own sexual functions and enjoyments. No woman is quite free from these early biases; for they are part of early life itself.

MATURATIONAL HURDLES

Two facts are important for us. The first is that, because of these early fantasies about maternal rivalry, vengefulness, or need for extra-devotion because of the daughter's sexuality, some degree of shame, guilt about offending mother, remorse, disgust or sense of impending punishment is inescapable at every new step in feminine development, no matter how permissive the world around her, and no matter what counterbalancing features of love, pride and joy she may have in achievement.

The second important fact concerns maturational crises. Growing girls suffer variously the many problems of growing up, yet by the time they are women many achieve in their daily lives fair control over, and commonsense adaptation to, these internal biases; but at critical maturational hurdles these controls are liable to fail dramatically. The early maternal fantasy relations acquire renewed force at puberty, at courtship, at consummation, at marriage, during pregnancy, at childbirth and in the puerperium, at lactation and at the menopause.

At each venture into territory that has so far been only her mother's, the girl's varying degrees of pride and pleasure at the identification with the approving early mother images are liable to be hampered by guilts and fears, apparently illogical but derived much from the other unconscious early images of the faithless, or damaged, or revengeful, or prostitute mother. Where the early developments have gone well minor disturbances of anxiety or loss of confidence can be expected, but when they have gone badly, severe disturbances resting on guilt, panic, and depression may appear at the developmental crises already mentioned.

DEALING WITH GUILT AND ANXIETY

Human beings deal with guilt and anxiety in different ways. Some try to defy and fight these feelings, bluff them out frantically, deny and disown self-disapproval within themselves and carry out deeds which they feel are forbidden and more or less delinquent; but we may notice how often by this flouted defiance they get others to be condemning about them so the condemnation is not abolished – merely redistributed. Others bravely seek out the very field which arouses anxiety in a struggle to act sensibly and be 'with it' and now overcome their sexual uneasiness in new ways. But the most common way of surmounting guilt about, or fear of, the early mother figure over sexual enjoyment is to limit the amount of feminine pleasure to dull, sober proportions.

Women with severe guilts renounce feminine joys and live more or less grimly or, worse still, lead lives of sexual suffering; all these in attempts to appease the asexual or forbidding or wounded or terrifying maternal figures which were internalized in childhood. Where such appeasements of forbidding internal figures and the consequent spoiling of femininity are insufficient to assuage guilts and terrors then these may break out as frankly emotional crises, usually of panics and depressions, at the various steps in feminine development.

Minor crises are the stuff of common family life which faces and copes with emotional difficulties in growing girls, courting women, young brides, young mothers, mothers of adolescents and menopausal women. Larger emotional crises are the stuff of the non-medical helping professions, school teachers, youth leaders, police, probation officers, social workers, the Samaritans, clergy, youth counsellors, solicitors, barmaids, health visitors, midwives, neighbours, relatives. Both mild and severe crises are met by obstetricians, GPs, paediatricians, and psychiatrists. Last, as we doctors know only too well, bodily sacrifices may also be offered, varying from dysmenorrhoea to vaginal anaesthesia or dyspareunia, from abortion to fearful and difficult labour, from horror at breastfeeding to secondary frigidity, from searches for sterilization to problems with all contraceptives, from menorrhagia to hysterectomy. The guilts and terrors so far outlined and the need to offer sacrifices are of course not the only possible causes of medical events in women, but they are often complicating causes and sometimes basic ones.

PUBERTY

With the major feminine step of puberty the upsurge of sexual longings, driven by the endocrines, brings an accompanying upsurge of the old guilts and fears which the child has more or less successfully repressed during her school years. These longings and the guilts and fears now take more sophisticated forms and are no longer associated only with parental figures, although they usually include them. The unconscious relation with the early mother figures can again be discerned in distorted beliefs which the girl now will hold, not only about her present mother, but also about other older women. The frigid, sweet madonna, the prostitute, the hateful, punishing witch, the reproachful, damaged mother, the jealous, resentful rival, etc., all reappear in her relations with older women, school teachers, neighbours, mothers and sisters, friends, public women, film stars and television figures. For example, the school teacher may be feared as a hateful punishing witch, her mother as reproachful, worn out and never to be left, the health visitor as a sweet, devoted madonna, the neighbour as a frigid, jealous and resentful rival, the brother's wife as a grasping prostitute.

There is always a grain of truth in these beliefs but all these figures get classified in pretty absolute terms on small and rarely corroborated evidence. It is of interest that these same figures can also be fairly easily noted – with all the emotional responses to them – at the other crises of marriage, pregnancy, labour, puerperium and during early motherhood, as well as, although less distinctly, at the menopause.

At her marriage, some older woman may be suspected as regarding her as too young (or too old) or marrying above (or below) her station, or being callous about leaving her poor mother just when she needs her. During pregnancy the 'old bag' across the street is felt as always peering at her through the curtains. In labour the young black nurse was an angel, but the ward nursing officer was an old witch who just enjoys women's sufferings and will not let them see their babies out of spite and jealousy.

Around the menopause the girls of today may be seen as sex mad, no sense of control, disgusting, and should be stopped. In such pictures it is sometimes not difficult to see the old early images in modern dress.

ADULT PROBLEMS

If we ignore the complicated developmental struggles of puberty and how these may be blighted when early developments have gone ill and turn to survey briefly other adult crises one matter is clear: some women – those who as infants grew a loving admiration for their mother's femininity – surmount the various crises of feminine development with relative ease. They anticipate eagerly and welcome each new development, and can confidently and sensibly ask their mothers and other helpers, as one grown woman among others, for tips and ideas over each new development, while retaining their own autonomy and dignity. They are not uneasy at owning their private sexual wishes and their private sexual parts and at learning without envy from the experience of others and they do not have to prove anything by being shamefully fabulous or super at sex, or at marriage, or at mothering. The less guilt the freer is enjoyment in all aspects of female sexual life, and the deeper and less frantic or defiant their pleasures. Such women can love and trust others without clinging dependence, and can co-operate gladly and gratefully but not subserviently with their men; and so with their babies (and incidentally with their obstetricians). Not only are they loving but they are lovable; truly they make love, for they bring out the loving side of others. If they disagree and quarrel they do so early and honestly without sulks or malice. And if they suffer losses they mourn with love but recover (eventually) without seeking to blame others or make them feel guilty.

Doctors, whose job is trouble, meet less than their fair share of such women, so it is useful to be reminded that they exist. To come down to earth, many women are capable of many of these states of mind, if their lives go well, but they are rarely absolute states, and like all achievements are usually a bit rocky, liable to come and go, and to be under strain at crises. The truly unfortunate women however rarely achieve them, but come to the fields of femininity more as lifelong trespassers, with guilts and fears of trouble, so that their lives as women are chancy and limited in greater or lesser degree. Many have difficulties in consummating their relationship with a man, and some girls cannot consummate at all and are even innocent of knowledge of their genital area. Some dare not touch it – and it seems for them to be still only dirty or the banned property of a sexually selfish mother who keeps all knowledge for herself. Some girls even say reproachfully,

'My mother never told me anything', as if the bookstalls and cinemas were not blatant with the facts of life, but also as if she is forbidden to know for herself and still resents her mother for not sharing her secrets. Other young women seem anxious to remain innocent children not only in knowledge but in physique, and to yield the field of womanhood to their grown up mothers; some of them seek to live with or near their mothers even after marriage; others may believe that their vaginas are too small for intercourse and that this will tear them apart (although it is remarkable how quickly many inherit their adulthood and their vaginas if a woman doctor can introduce them to their vaginas).

Some can have a sexual life only so long as it is young and guilt-laden and irresponsible but once committed to marriage have to retreat from joy and become frigid, unable because of old, wicked rivalry to become happily married women. Others become frigid only after childbirth – because mothers are madonnas. Some frigid girls simply avoid marriage with its rivalry of mother and live in respectable but unsatisfied sin, while others, unable to enjoy any aspect of sex, rush into marriage hoping desperately that its respectability will take away their sense of sin about sexuality and magically cure them of pre-marital frigidity. Others are able to enjoy intercourse fully only if contraceptive precautions are absent or unreliable, so that they can enjoy the fantasy that they do it essentially to get babies. Many honeymoons and later marital pleasures are wrecked by guilt-driven frigidity; sex is cruel, painful, or dirty and disgusting, or animal-like – unless it is for babies. Suffering by being too tired or having a headache at the prospect of bed is all too well-known. Certain women can enjoy intercourse fully only after provoking and suffering a painful row or a beating which can assuage their guilt for the time being. Others create rows the next day to atone for the wickedness of the night before. Many is the child who dreads Sundays because that is the day for the parents to quarrel.

Friendly encouragement and goodwill from others that she should enjoy her man, together with patience and love from a husband who is confident of his masculinity, are needed by many women to counteract this sense of guilt; but when the guilt is massive no reassurances are effective: indeed the woman may regard her husband and other encouragers only as evil-minded tempters requiring her to commit disgusting acts of concupiscence.

Going further and permanently into womanhood and actually bearing a child can be the greatest trespass of all. Maternity, the peak achievement of sexual growth, tests the whole early system of the mother/girl relationship and it carries the greatest potential of all for arousing the rages and reproaches of the internalized mother. Where the guilt-laden woman was liable to be anxious or frigid or hostile about intercourse, she will have related feelings about pregnancy. Where she was docile, obedient and clingingly anxious to please mother over her marriage, she will now show related anxious obedience at antenatal classes and procedures but will not decide for herself nor be adventurous.

Fears of miscarriage; expectation of punitively painful child-birth; labour as a fearful experience in which she can lose her life or her baby's; and many problems over enjoying the baby after-wards arise out of unconscious guilt feelings towards the early mother. Far from enjoying her baby she may be afraid of or averse to him, unable to own him fiercely as her own. Some may even seek her mother or some other woman to adopt the baby and they thereby surrender their motherhood altogether. Advice to enjoy the baby is difficult for such young mothers to listen to but they are all too vulnerable to criticisms about their various incompetences with the baby. It must be admitted that young mothers rarely lack advisers but only those who are confident of their rights to be mothers can view these advisers as helpful and rather envying assistants, rather than harassing and hostile parents to be disobeyed at peril.

And so on. Throughout adult womanhood the internalized relation to the early maternal figure has major influence on whether or not the wife and mother copes gladly and confidently with each new development task or has to feel guilt, depression, timidity and anxiety; and whether she feels internally free and supported or alone, unblessed, criticized. For other tasks lie ahead of her. Can she enjoy her body and her baby as a wife and mother? Can she build a family, a home? Can she rejoice in her husband's masculinity, strength and successes? Can she continue to feel loved by, and loving towards, her older mother? Can she be glad to be a 40-year-old woman, sexually, domestically, soci-ally? Does she experience both regret and pride as her children grow up and can she be glad to be their mother? Can she welcome her own daughter's menstruation, and be friendly to this new rival's growing interest in sexuality? Or will the old rivalries now lead her to anger, the old jealousies to sulks, the old envies to destructiveness? Can she accept with admiration the younger generation which begins to take over as the repository of sexual femininity – just as her mother was in her childhood? Will she admire them for it as she once admired her mother, or will she feel she herself is again too sexy and must renounce all sexual interest and feel jealous of the younger generation, bitter and discarded once again? And what when her daughter has babies; and her daughter-in-law?

All these are hurdles of development; potentially enriching experiences but liable to be tormenting because of the biases mentioned earlier and their accompanying rages, envies, fears of criticism, and depressions.

And now the menopause and the loss of the capacity to have babies. Will it revive old infantile rages and hatreds at the sexual vigour of the women who can have babies, with wishes to spoil and filthy up their joys; or will it be accepted with love and goodwill and admiration of these others? Will she become an admiring grandmother, glad to be a minor assistant to the new vigorous adults? Or will she be interfering, invalid, jealous, spoiler, bitter, reproachful and lonely.

The answers to these questions will be much based upon how the woman fared in the inevitable earlier experiences, real and fantasized, with her own mother years ago.

And now, to redress the inevitable distortion of emphasis which arises from the selection for examination of any single aspect of female development, it needs mention that many influences other than the early relation with the mother will promote or mar the development of femininity. The relation to the father is an obvious one, especially in fashioning later relations to men. The luck of brothers or sisters, of friends and aunts and uncles and grand-mothers, or early health and illness, and, above these, the actual relations between the parents are obviously also important. But behind all of these is the early primary, fantasy-ridden relation with the mother and the child's inevitable struggles with love and hatred of her in this first relation of all.

12

Discharges and irritations in psychosexual medicine

H. M. Bramley

SUMMARY

- The unstructured interview: what is told
- The genital examination: what is revealed
- The doctor/patient interaction
- Unrealistic ideas: unmasked, understood and uprooted

Most complaints of genital discharge have a physiological or pathological cause, but a few are a cover up for other distresses. Some pathological discharges precipitate or exacerbate already existing psychosexual problems. Complaints of genital discharge, presented in whatever setting, must of course have an appropriate history taken and suitable tests performed to exclude physical disease or injury. If these tests prove negative it is considered good practice to repeat them. If the results are still negative, the doctor has to decide if the complaint or distress has emotional roots which should be sought. Sometimes the words used to describe physical sensations can be seen to be symbolic of the patient's feelings. Such words as 'pain', 'soreness' and 'irritation' can apply to emotions as well as to bodily symptoms, and may provide a key to unspoken, and often unrecognized, emotional troubles. The doctor who can listen and think about the words used may be able to make more sense of the situation. However, a direct interpretation to the patient may not be appropriate especially early in the consultation. The emotion has probably been suppressed by the patient because acknowledgement would be too painful, and expression in the form of a physical symptom is easier. The following cases illustrate some of these problems and indicate the outcomes.

> Mrs A, a smartly dressed, capable woman in her early 40s complained to her doctor about a vaginal discharge and irritation. The doctor examined her and found no evidence of abnormal discharge or other pathology. He took all the appropriate tests, which turned out to be negative. She persisted in returning time after time over a period of more than two years. The doctor carefully explained each time that he could find nothing wrong and reassured her that she was perfectly healthy. Finally, she complained no more about discharge but developed a more bizarre symptom, saying that after sexual intercourse with her husband she had panic attacks which left her debilitated for days, and this had forced her to stop having sex with him altogether. The GP felt this was beyond his province, and so referred her to a psychosexual clinic. The doctor there discovered that her sex life with her husband had been very unsatisfactory, and she had felt used rather than loved. This had been a reflection of their whole life together throughout their marriage of 20 years, which had included bringing up three children. With this persistent and distressing discharge and irritation, Mrs A had hoped that her irritation with her husband would be discovered and helped. Sadly, for years her real distress was never discussed and she was too shy to mention it openly. By the time she was referred for further help she had made a commitment elsewhere with the resultant upset of family life.

When patients display persistent, illogical behaviour they are often trying unconsciously to get help for an unhappy area of their lives. Patients choose the person to whom they will take their troubles for their own reasons; they may not be conscious of why they have made this choice. Those with a complaint of genital discharge may appear at the doctor's surgery, may insist on being sent to a gynaecologist, may attend family planning or well women clinics, or may choose the department of genito-urinary medicine (GUM) depending on what the patient feels about herself and what she hopes to receive from the doctor. Mrs A brought her discharge and irritation to her GP, no doubt because she felt he was the person who could help her with her unhappy life, although too shy to tell him the real reason. Perhaps she was not fully conscious of it herself.

THE UNSTRUCTURED INTERVIEW: WHAT IS TOLD

Mrs B, who had never had extra-marital exposure, chose the GUM clinic first of all because she felt it was appropriate for her complaint. She attended not once but many times and in different towns. All the tests done had been negative, although she complained of a discharge and was sure she had a venereal disease. The doctors had reassured her many times that she had nothing to worry about. Reassurance proved to be of little use as no one had discovered what Mrs B's real anxiety was.

Mrs B sat down at the desk of another GUM physician. She was dressed in girlish clothes, and looked much younger than her years. She said, 'I'm sure I've got a venereal disease which is giving me a discharge and irritation. I can't have sex with my husband in case I might infect him, and he's cross with me now as we haven't had sex for so long.' Instead of doing the usual history taking and testing for sexually transmitted disease, the doctor, who had noted the years of negative tests, looked at what was happening in the present relationship between himself and the patient. He noted that the girl – or so she presented herself although five years married – was begging advice from him in a child-to-authority manner. He commented, 'You seem to expect me to be a sort of parent who can solve all your problems.' The girl then said, 'It's my parents who are the problem.' She always felt that as the eldest child in the family her parents had expected more of her in conduct and good performance than she could manage.

When she was 15 years old she had behaved very badly by encouraging the next-door neighbour, who had interfered with her sexually, and actually allowing him once to have sexual intercourse with her. She had deceived her parents and felt that she was having her just reward now by having some sort of foul disease, which was giving her the discharge. She had a firmly-rooted idea that disobedience to and deception of parents brings on venereal disease or some sort of appropriate punishment. After a lengthy discussion she seemed able to understand her need to punish herself, and later understood the need to forgive herself. Mrs B realized that she need no longer rely on her parents precepts, but could now make her own moral decisions. The continual tests for venereal disease were not now necessary as there had been no extra-marital exposure with either partner. She attended the clinic once more for a further discussion with the doctor, who was pleased she was having happy sexual intercourse with her husband.

When a patient presents at a GUM clinic with fear of, or symptoms connected with, sexually transmitted disease, a full history and appropriate sets of investigations must of course be done. When all are repeatedly negative and there is no history of extra-marital exposure, then a different approach is necessary. This patient chose this clinic because her fantasy was that she had a justly deserved venereal affliction.

History taking would only have produced the same information as before. Mrs B had never mentioned in previous visits to the clinic this episode in her adolescence of which she was ashamed. The important facts only emerged when the doctor commented on what was taking place between the doctor and the patient at the present moment, and allowed the patient to say what she wanted. Facts did not emerge with questioning. The doctor would never have thought of asking about sexual abuse by a much older neighbour. An unstructured interview with a comment on how the patient was behaving made it easier for the patient to say what was really bothering her. She was not told that her fantasy was ridiculous and unrealistic, and she was not reassured yet again that her discharge was normal; she was helped to understand why she was punishing herself. Then she could make a decision for herself whether she could now abandon her fantasy and have a more realistic attitude to her sexuality.

THE GENITAL EXAMINATION: WHAT IS REVEALED

Patients who present with a complaint of genital discharge need of course to have a genital examination. This examination can give a lot of physical information, but for those interested in psychosexual medicine it can yield a great deal more information of a different kind. The man who presents with a urethral discharge may say as the doctor asks him to drop his pants for examination and tests, 'I'm afraid I've always been smaller than everyone else down there.' When the doctor examines him, he finds genitals within a perfectly normal range of size. What does this statement unconsciously mean for the patient as a man? Does he feel unable to compete with other men for women's attention, or does he feel he somehow cannot satisfy his wife properly? This sort of anxiety is again usually a fantasy. The man himself, if given space, will tell the doctor what it means, and then, incidentally, he may receive help with an emotional problem as well as treatment for his discharge.

The woman too, when being examined for complaint of discharge, may complain she is too small and an examination may hurt her, or she may demonstrate this sort of idea about herself by tightening her vaginal muscles and making the examination difficult. Is she telling the doctor she is too small to have sexual intercourse, and does that mean she does not feel mature enough for the responsibilities of a wife and mother? Perhaps it means she is angry and keeping the doctor out, as she may be keeping her husband out if she thinks he has given her the discharge, or for any other angry reason. She may feel her discharge is too dirty to be examined. The doctor will not know the answer until the patient tells him, and, there may then be more work to do beyond that of just diagnosing and treating the original complaint. When patients are in this vulnerable position of genital examination, they may often expose what feelings and ideas they have about themselves and their sexual functioning if this is disturbing them or is unsatisfactory in some way.

Miss C, a bright, plump, pretty girl, was sent to a psychosexual clinic by a gynaecologist because she had com-

plained of having a discharge of which he had found no
evidence, and of being unable to have sexual intercourse with her partner of some years standing. When
she attended the clinic she was dressed in black, as
though she was mourning the loss of her partner. She
had sent him away since her interview with the gynaecologist because she was afraid he would ask for sex,
and she knew she had a discharge and that she was
abnormal 'down below'. The fact that she had been
reassured that all was perfectly normal had made no
difference to her. The doctor asked her to get on to the
couch for examination. While the doctor was very gently
and slowly putting his finger into the patient's vagina,
it seemed to open the door to a torrent of information
which had never been revealed before.

She had had a relationship with her uncle when she
was ten years old. She used to go to his house after
school as both her parents and her aunt worked full
time. Her uncle did night work but was awake by the
time she arrived from school. They were fond of each
other. It began by a little touching, and progressed over
the period of about a year to him putting the tip of his
penis into her vaginal opening. He did not hurt her, but
she felt it was wrong, yet wondered if this was what all
uncles did, as he had tried to make her feel it was normal
and natural. She did not tell her mother as she thought
she would not believe her. Miss C felt there was something wrong with her genital area now because of these
episodes in the past. The evidence of this was her discharge, and the fact that she had been unable to have
sexual intercourse, although she had tried on two
occasions. When the doctor finished the examination,
during which he had received all this information, he
had found nothing abnormal except very slight tightening of the vaginal muscles and a clear, normal discharge. The doctor suggested that the feelings of
damage might be to herself as a sexual person rather
than to her actual genitals. The patient said she felt
angry and affronted that her uncle should treat her in
this way and then pretend it had never happened. She
said loudly that she would never forgive him unless he
apologized. She still went to visit her uncle and aunt,

and when a programme about child sexual abuse came on to the television she wanted to shout in a loud voice, 'That's what you did to me.' She shared a lot of her anger with the doctor, and asked him if she should confront her uncle with it and tell him how angry she was. She feared that if she did her uncle would deny it all, or that he would have a heart attack as he had only recently had one. The doctor said she was no longer a girl and must decide for herself what to do.

After four interviews and a gap of six months, Miss C bounced in, beaming from ear to ear, brightly and prettily dressed. She said things were fine now; she had met another boy three months ago and they had recently had intercourse. She had enjoyed it, was very happy with him, and hoped it would be a permanent relationship. She had not confronted her uncle, but had talked quite a lot about it to her mother and one of her aunts. Miss C had overcome her conflict of loving her uncle and perhaps enjoying the closeness she had with him, and hating what he did to her and his pretence of forgetting it. She felt that the damage he had done had been repaired now that she had had successful sex with her new partner.

An unstructured interview had been essential so that Miss C could tell the doctor her story and talk about her conflicting ambivalent feelings towards her uncle. Even though the interview was unstructured, the vital information that was so private did not emerge until her private parts were being examined. This opened the door for Miss C to talk about her fantasy of damage both to her vagina and to herself, being treated as an object which her uncle used without apology, instead of treating her as a loved niece. She came to accept there was no physical damage when the doctor encouraged her to examine herself, but it took her longer to come to terms with her angry feelings about how she had been treated, and the guilty feelings about her part in it.

THE DOCTOR/PATIENT INTERACTION

In psychosexual medicine, being aware of what is going on in the drama being played out between doctor and patient, and trying to understand why the two produce a certain sort of atmosphere can give the doctor indications of what the real problem is for the patient. The disturbance may be hidden in the patient's unconscious mind and initially hidden from the doctor, although clues can be given from the way the patient is behaving in the consultation. The sensitive time of the genital examination, which of course must always be performed with a complaint of discharge, can often give indicators as to the nature of the disturbance in the patient's life, as in the following case.

Miss D, a 24-year-old typist, went to her GP and complained of a discharge causing soreness. Swabs showed *Candida albicans* infection. Suitable treatment was given, but the patient kept coming back with complaints of soreness. Swabs thereafter were negative. She finally said, 'I can't make love with my boyfriend.' The doctor sent her to a psychosexual clinic, where she complained of inability to permit sexual intercourse because she was frightened of being hurt. The doctor expected that on vaginal examination she would find a protective vaginismus because of the pain that a thrush vaginitis can cause. To her surprise, the examination was easy as the patient had not experienced difficulty when using Tampax. The doctor noticed a marked look of disgust on the patient's face as she did the examination and thought that the girl felt disgust about her genitals. The doctor was wrong again, as the patient and her boyfriend enjoyed mutual masturbation, and when the patient was asked to explore her own painful vagina, she did so without difficulty. It is always unwise to make assumptions in psychosexual work, as the answer is so often different from what one expects.

What then was the look of disgust, and what was the fear of pain related to? The doctor and patient puzzled over this, and the girl eventually related that when she was 16 she had gone out with a man much older than herself who she liked and trusted. When he asked for intercourse with her she had been very reluctant, but he at last persuaded her on the promise that if it was hurting her he would stop at once. What happened next was a rapid and forceful penetration while she screamed at him to stop. It gave her a terrible fright, as well as misery because he had broken his promise. She found out later he was having sex with a number of girls, and particularly liked 'breaking in' virgins. She was disgusted with herself for allowing herself to be used as a plaything.

She kept returning to the doctor and talking about the trauma of this episode, apologizing that she had not yet managed intercourse, although consciously she very much wanted to achieve it. The doctor noticed she was relating to her like a naughty schoolgirl who had not done her homework, and a comment about this to the patient prompted the girl to talk about her parents, who she loved, and to express the feeling that perhaps she was not quite ready to leave home. Finally, after nearly two years of sporadic interviews, she appeared full of smiles saying she was now living with her boyfriend, they had planned their wedding, and that intercourse had been achieved.

The start of work with this girl was the look of disgust on her face, which was only shown during the vaginal examination, not when she sat dressed in the chair. Only the patient had the answer to that look of disgust, and not until she talked about it did she realize how strongly the memory of the traumatic episode had affected her. The way in which the girl put the doctor into a parental role enabled the doctor to make a comment, and this forced the patient to look at feelings she had not been conscious of before.

UNREALISTIC IDEAS: UNMASKED, UNDERSTOOD AND UPROOTED

Part of the work of psychosexual medicine is helping patients to express their fantasies or the unrealistic ideas they have about their sexual abilities and functioning. Fantasies can be a block to a patient's ability to lead a normal, happy sex life with their partner. When they have been expressed, they must be treated seriously, no matter how bizarre, because they are part of a patient's feelings about herself and her sexual functioning. When the patient has been able to realize the symbolic truth about the fantasy, and to compare the actual idea, which is not compatible with reality, then she can discard it. She is then able to deal with its symbolic meaning. Mrs P had done this when she gave up the idea that sexual misdemeanours and deceiving parents results in venereal disease as retribution.

> Mrs E, a 29-year-old housewife, attended a GUM clinic with the fear that because she had had extra-marital intercourse her present discharge might be the sign of some sexually transmitted disease. Her husband, who was returning from a business trip, would want sex when he returned, and she was afraid he would find out about her behaviour. The tests were positive for gonorrhoea. Mrs T completed the course of treatment before her husband returned, and her extra-marital partner was also found and treated. Four years later she complained to the health visitor that she was always tense and cross and shouting at her children. She also complained that she felt abnormal because she never wanted sex with her husband. She was referred to a psychosexual clinic.
>
> Mrs E was a pretty, talkative woman who told the doctor she never wanted sex, but that her husband wanted it every night. She then said she really did want it, but the feeling was all locked inside her. She talked on and on, giving the doctor no clues as to the cause of her difficulty, and perhaps trying to fend off the vaginal examination. When the doctor did at last suggest this, the patient said she was dirty and therefore could not be examined. The doctor looked at her clean fresh dress and asked when she had last had a bath. The patient said yesterday, so the doctor persuaded her to get on to the couch, meanwhile wondering what the 'dirty' really meant. While the examination was taking place, the patient said her brother had complained that it was like having sex 'in a big pail' after his wife had had a baby. Mrs E said she felt she was abnormal down below, and perhaps her vagina was also like a pail, although her last pregnancy had been five years ago. The doctor invited her to feel inside her vagina, and she said that it felt quite normal, although that was not what she had expected. The doctor was then left to puzzle out the

meaning of these two fantasies about the vagina, that it was 'dirty' and that it was like a 'big pail'.

When patients complain that their vagina is too big it sometimes indicates they have a capacity for sex that is greater than they feel is legitimate, or that they can handle. The doctor felt it was the opposite with this patient, however, as she did not seem to want sexual intercourse. He felt helpless and stupid that he could not work this out, and felt vulnerable and unable to help the patient. He confessed to the patient that he could not understand what the dirty vagina and the big pail meant. The patient started crying and told him about the extra-marital affair she had had with a married man and that she had been treated for gonorrhoea without her husband's knowledge. It was against all her principles, and she felt very guilty about it. The doctor was then able to share with the patient the symbolic meanings of the dirty vagina and the big pail, which she accepted. She returned to say they had started having sex again, but she couldn't really abandon herself in enjoyment as she knew she was able to reach several climaxes, and her husband might want to know where she had learnt this! She was still feeling that her capacity for sex was greater than was proper, as symbolized by the 'big pail'.

Another type of fantasy related to sex but not to the genitals was mentioned by Mr F, a married man who came to the GUM clinic with a urethral discharge, which was diagnosed as non-specific urethritis. He had repeated attacks over about two years. When asked about his extra-marital sexual contacts, he admitted they had been men, as he was bisexual. On one attendance at the clinic he was very distressed and the doctor listened to a tale of his wife's fear of catching AIDS from him and her refusal to have sexual intercourse. As he was talking about sex with his wife the doctor noticed that Mr F was doing so in a furtive sort of way without looking at him. The doctor remarked that the patient seemed to feel that sex was a very indecent subject to discuss, which brought the rejoinder, 'Well, it is, isn't it? Women have to put up with it because chaps have to have it.' In the course of conversation about this he revealed a traumatic tale of adolescent sexual abuse, and stated firmly that sex was only a strong instinct that needed release, and that women were never very interested in it. This fantasy that sex is only for men was changed when later he discovered that his wife always had to masturbate after sex because she felt so frustrated by his deliberately quick method of having intercourse. His change in attitude to his wife and her sex needs was very marked after he was able to accept that sex might be good and right between married people, and not the furtive, necessary release for a man he had thought it to be. Their sex life greatly improved, and was regular and mostly satisfactory. Although occasional urges remained to attend a sauna, which would give him male contact, Mr F was able to resist them because sex at home had been discussed openly, with resultant improvement in frequency and quality. His fantasy about his sexual self was that men are beasts who have to have a sexual outlet; his childhood experiences had never allowed him to think of sex in a loving, constructive context.

A final case may illustrate some of the ways already mentioned in which a doctor is given clues about a patient's sexual problem by the way in which the patient unconsciously communicates signs of the distress lying behind the complaint of discharge.

Mrs G complained of a discharge to the health visitor, who had called upon her to examine her two-month-old baby. The health visitor advised her to go to the GUM clinic, which she dutifully did. All the tests were negative, and no one suspected she had any further troubles. She tried again to get help by attending her GP, with a complaint of pain down below, discharge, and difficulty with sexual intercourse. The patient told him that all her GUM tests had been negative. The doctor noticed she was wearing very loose clothes, which hid her good figure. He enquired what the difficulty was, and the patient said she still had pain on intercourse, and she thought she had been torn during the birth of her baby, who was now nine months old. He asked her to get ready for an examination, and was aware she did this very slowly and with great reluctance. She eventually sat up on the couch, knees under her chin and arms clasped tightly round her legs. As the doctor approached the couch, he had a strong feeling that it would be indecent to examine this woman – and then realized that this feeling was coming from the patient. He remarked that it seemed very difficult for Mrs G to allow an examination, whereupon she said that sex had never been very successful in her marriage.

When she eventually straightened her legs, the doctor noticed a Caesarean section scar. A quick look at the perineum revealed no tear, and yet the patient was complaining of painful sexual intercourse. The doctor asked what the idea of being torn could mean, as the woman had been delivered by Caesarean section and this was her first child. The patient responded with a long story about how, although not very successful with sex, she was determined to be the perfect mother. She had attended all the prenatal classes and read all the books, but when the moment came her husband was banished, an anaesthetic administered, and a Caesarean section took place. She felt a terrible failure as a woman, and her idea of herself as the perfect mother had been 'torn up'.

At the next visit, the patient said she felt much happier and the pain below had gone, but she still had not been able to have intercourse. The doctor remembered her slowness to get on the couch and her reluctance to be examined, and saw that although she was neatly and well dressed, her clothes again camouflaged her good figure. The doctor asked how she felt about sexual intercourse now that the pain was gone. There was silence while the patient looked at her hands. The doctor tried to get her to say something about her relationship with her husband, but there was no response. After waiting a while, the doctor remarked that the patient expected him to do all the work – was this how she acted with her husband in intercourse? This freed the patient to say she did not feel she deserved to enjoy sex. At 13 she had gone on a skiing holiday with a school party. There was also a party of schoolboys in the chalet. She had been caught by one of her teachers being kissed and hugged by an Austrian boy. A great fuss was made about this, and she was labelled as being 'easy'. The reputation spread beyond her school to her village at home. She was mortified, and hated the joking remarks made to her. Shortly after this, she introduced her father to one of her school friend's mothers when being fetched from a party. This started a relationship, which resulted in many fierce and acrimonious quarrels between her mother and father. She felt that all the unhappiness in her home was due entirely to her. She had a fantasy that sexuality brings disaster. It took a number of sessions for her to come to terms with these feelings and ideas. She did finally allow her sexuality to come out, and eventually had another baby born the normal way.

The method of referral of this patient is interesting as it shows her determination to find help for her unsatisfactory sex life. Mrs G had to go by way of the health visitor, the GUM clinic, and to her GP for the help she needed. This must have been difficult for her as she was a shy woman. The doctor used the atmosphere created between them to pinpoint the patient's problems, first on the couch, by noting her 'fending-off' behaviour, and then by commenting on her silence and that perhaps she was letting him do all the work. The genital examination was appropriate and very important, as without it the doctor might never have discovered she had had a Caesarean section, and her feelings of failure as a mother, which were symbolized by the 'torn' vagina.

Fantasies about discharges, irritations, and the genital area in general have to be recognized for what they are – beliefs held by the patient that do not fit the obvious facts. They may be unconscious statements of what the patient really feels but of which she is not consciously aware. This patient's two fantasies were respected and constructively used to find out what the tearing meant, and why she did not deserve to enjoy sex. Reassurance that her vagina was intact would have been of no help to Mrs G, she had to understand the meaning of her 'torn' vagina, and to mourn her loss of becoming a perfect mother before she could accept sex again. Her fantasy of not deserving sexual pleasure and its cause had to be acknowledged, understood, and uprooted before she could fully enjoy sex for the first time.

Most men and women complaining of genital discharge are competently managed by the standard approach of classical medicine: history, examination, differential diagnosis, special tests, diagnosis and treatment. The purpose of this chapter is to illustrate that psychosexual problems may be linked to a pathological, physiological, or imagined discharge. These matters may be of great personal importance, and are unlikely to be uncovered or helped by the classical medical approach; bland reassurance helps the doctor only. Alertness to the possibility of deeper problems is of primary importance. The cases quoted, although much abbreviated, give some indication of the often tortuous and bizarre fantasies which need to be discovered, examined, and dealt with. They also illustrate the importance of active listening, of observing vital clues that may be offered in a genital examination, and of a continuous sensitivity to what is taking place between doctor and patient.

13

Pelvic pain and dyspareunia

H. Montford

SUMMARY

- Physical causes
- The problems of physical investigation and treatment
- Physical symptoms as a remembrance of times past
- Pain as a 'visiting card'
- Physical symptoms as an expression of emotional pain

'I've got this pain, doctor, and when we make love it hurts.' Inherent in this statement lies a need for body/mind doctoring. The patient is seeking a doctor, one who will examine and investigate, diagnose and treat her pain. The patient is also revealing an emotional part of her life – making love – which is being disturbed and threatened by the pain. Such patients are an important part of the work of doctors trained in psychosexual medicine.

The patient may go first of all to her general practitioner, or she may choose a family planning clinic where the freedom to talk about sexual matters is expected and accepted. The patient may have been referred to a department of gynaecology or genito-urinary medicine. A psychosexually trained doctor may work in any of these settings. Here there is the unique opportunity to examine the genital parts and to arrange for investigation and treatment as necessary, while seeing the patient as a whole person and looking for the existence and cause of any emotional pain.

Alternatively, the patient may already have had physical investigations which have revealed no organic cause for the complaint, and has then been referred to a doctor working as a specialist in a psychosexual problems clinic. The doctor's work will depend on the setting in which the patient is seen. However, if body and mind can be looked at together from the beginning, much time and trouble may be saved, and further pain to the patient may be avoided.

PHYSICAL CAUSES

Any complaint of pain that could possibly have a physical cause must be properly investigated, and it would be a brave or foolhardy doctor indeed who failed to observe this. It is not within the scope of this chapter to give details of such physical investigations nor of conditions found. The diagnosis of pelvic pain, while still an enigma to gynaecologists, has to a large extent been revolutionized by the use of ultrasound and laparoscope. The increasing use of technology will no doubt elicit further demonstrable causes of pelvic pain. Nevertheless, it is known that a physical sign does not necessarily have at its root a physical disorder. One can compare the pain of migraine, which may be shown to be due to dilatation of the cerebral arteries, while the cause of the migraine is often due to stress. Similarly, the dilatation of pelvic veins may not be due to structural disease but can have an emotional cause, although the mechanism by which this occurs is likewise ill-understood. Research will again lead to further knowledge and understanding of the relationship between symptoms, demonstrable physical signs, and emotional factors.

> Miss P had been under a gynaecologist for eight months for pelvic pain. X-rays had shown dilated veins in her pelvis, and she had been given large doses of a hormone, which she said made her fat and irritable. The pain was no better. She had stopped seeing the gynaecologist, and was hoping the family planning doctor could help.
> Miss P was plump and pretty and looked much

younger than her 24 years. She chatted about her mum, who was really worried for her. Her sisters were all older and married and seemed to be all right. She had had no problem until she had left home in the north and come to live with her boyfriend in London. The doctor said she must miss her mum being so far away. Miss P's eyes filled with tears as she said yes, she did, but she loved her boyfriend too and wanted to be with him.

The doctor noticed her feelings of reluctance to suggest a pelvic examination, feeling this 'little girl' had been through many examinations already. Miss P, however, said it was all right, she did not mind, but she hoped the doctor would be gentle as she was rather small inside.

The doctor's feelings about Miss P being so young and vulnerable were a reflection of Miss P's feelings about herself. This was confirmed by her belief that her vagina was too small, that is, not yet mature enough for sexual intercourse. By allowing Miss P to talk rather than by taking a history, the doctor was able firstly to understand Miss P's feelings about being the baby of the family, and, secondly, that the pelvic pain began only when she moved away from home and went to live with her boyfriend.

During pelvic examination which revealed a completely normal vagina, the doctor encouraged Miss P to talk about what being 'small' meant to her. She also encouraged her to feel inside her own vagina, to know its actual size for herself.

By the second interview Miss P had had intercourse on two occasions without pain. She had discussed the future with her boyfriend, and had made some adult decisions about buying a flat together, and perhaps eventually moving back to the north. The doctor found she already felt less protective towards Miss P, and even suggested that she return to the gynaecologist for another pelvic venogram, but unfortunately Miss P refused.

In this case, while not denying the existence of pelvic pathology, it was understanding and interpreting Miss P's feelings about herself that enabled her to relax and allow herself to enjoy intercourse without pain.

THE PROBLEMS OF PHYSICAL INVESTIGATION AND TREATMENT

For some patients with pelvic pain, the exclusion of a physical cause may come as an immense emotional relief with subsequent relief from pain. Fear of cancer or damage to the pelvic organs from childbirth or from disease may lead to muscle tension with consequent dyspareunia. Reassurance without exploring the fantasy, however, is not enough.

A woman was convinced she had cancer of the womb. She refused to accept the doctor's assurance that all was completely normal and there was no evidence of disease. Finally, she admitted to feeling a lump in her vagina, which was tender and intercourse made it more so. The doctor was able to show her that what she was feeling was her cervix, and that the sensation she was experiencing was the tenderness of pleasure, not pain.

For other patients the investigations or the treatment itself – particularly when painful, intrusive, or mutilating – may further increase or even be the cause of more persistent pain. When finally referred to the psychosexual doctor, such patients often bring much rage and anguish at being dismissed as disturbed, hypochondriacal, hysterical, or attention-seeking. The psychosexually trained doctor does not react, does not offer reassurance, but accepts these feelings as part of the patient's complaint. By allowing the patient to talk, by sharing with her the feelings of distress, and by using the twin tools of studying the doctor/patient relationship and the genital examination the real cause of the complaint may be discovered.

> Mrs J, aged 45, was referred to the psychosexual clinic by a gynaecologist. She was sent an appointment but did not reply nor attend. In his letter the gynaecologist said she had been attending his clinic for five years for pelvic pain. Mrs J had been given hormonal treatment, and finally her ovaries had been removed. She was now refusing intercourse as it made the pain worse. She had had a hysterectomy at age 28 in another part of the country.
>
> Another appointment was sent to Mrs J, this time enclosing a letter from the doctor encouraging her to come. Mrs J came, sullen, resentful, and half an hour late. The doctor was annoyed, but recognized that Mrs J's failure to keep appointments might be a symptom

of the problem. The doctor began by saying, 'You seem to have had a lot of treatment over the years but none of it has helped. You must be feeling pretty fed up with it.' A short silence. 'You didn't want to come, did you?' said the doctor. A torrent of rage poured out. How terrible it was to be a woman! Men didn't understand, they only made things worse! She had always had painful periods; she used to be kept at home in bed. Mrs J was brought up by mother and grandmother, father having left home when she was seven. When her periods stopped her mother took her to the doctor; 'The examination was awful. I know they thought I was pregnant, but how could I have been? I was never allowed a boyfriend.'

Eventually she married, a kind and patient man who did not trouble her too much, but a very difficult pregnancy and childbirth followed by extreme menorrhagia only confirmed her belief that mother and grandmother were right, and that being a woman was a terrible cross she had to bear. When a hysterectomy was suggested as the only means of cure, Mrs J accepted willingly, only to feel robbed of a chance of further pregnancies and permanently crippled as a woman.

By accepting this patient's rage the doctor was able to help Mrs J to understand that her anger was directed not so much at men as at mother and grandmother, who had brought her up to believe that feminine feelings and functions were shameful, burdensome, and should be hidden away. Sadly, however, although there was some improvement in Mrs J's appearance and manner, and intercourse was resumed, the feeling of irretrievable loss of her uterus and ovaries was too great to allow her to wholly relinquish her pain.

PHYSICAL SYMPTOMS AS A REMEMBRANCE OF TIMES PAST

For some patients a physical disorder of the genital organs, particularly if persistent and not responding easily to treatment, may be a reminder of past feelings about their bodies. Continuing vaginal soreness and discharge following an attack of thrush, when all swabs have long proved negative and appropriate medication no longer has the desired effect, may occur because the original infection confirmed in the patient's subconscious feelings that these parts, and therefore sex, is distasteful, dirty, disallowed, and therefore punishable. Unresolved anxieties about parental prohibition of sex, inadequacy as a sexual partner, ambivalence about an abortion, or past sexual abuse are all areas of feelings that can underly a complaint of pain.

> Margaret, a 40-year-old secretary, was plump and attractive, with smart, bright clothes and a fixed, bright smile. It was her second marriage; they had good jobs, no worries, and were extremely happy – but sex was painful. It was all because of a Bartholin's abscess in the vagina some years before; it must have left a scar because she could show the doctor exactly where it hurt. It was as if further discussion were unnecessary; this was a physical matter requiring physical examination only. Margaret undressed rapidly, chatting as she did so, climbed on the couch, readily separated her labia, and pointed to the painful area. Although she winced at first as the doctor touched it, she was able to tolerate vaginal examination easily. There was nothing abnormal to be seen or felt. The doctor recognized this woman's defences – that she was being 'put off'. She wanted to reassure her that all was normal; instead, still on the couch, she allowed her to talk.
>
> 'Perhaps I should stop the Pill,' said Margaret. 'I don't suppose I need it. I think I'm too old for babies now.' There was a pause. 'And that's sad for you,' said the doctor. 'Not really. . .' Another pause. 'I did get pregnant once. Oh, it was stupid and silly. It wasn't my husband, he didn't mean anything to me. I didn't believe in abortion but it was the only way. The day I went into hospital I started bleeding and suddenly it was all there in the bed, something in a mass of blood. It was awful.' Tears welled up in Margaret's eyes. 'And you haven't been able to forget?' asked the doctor. 'I thought I had, and then I had this abscess. It was so painful. On the day I went to the doctor it burst – there was blood. It brought it all back. It's never felt the same since. I really shouldn't have been so stupid.' 'And you have to punish yourself

for being stupid?' 'Silly, isn't it?' said Margaret, and smiled.

Four weeks later Margaret came again, looking much softer. 'It's all right now,' she said. 'I talked to my husband. I couldn't stop crying. He's never seen me like that. Then we made love and it didn't hurt at all.'

In confessing the past to the doctor and then to her husband, Margaret was able to accept her 'silliness' at becoming pregnant, and her guilt at wanting an abortion, which in the end proved inevitable.

PAIN AS A 'VISITING CARD'

All doctors are aware that their patients' presented complaint may not be the real reason for their visit. Particularly is this true in psychosexual medicine. Although we live in an age of sexual explicitness where the act of intercourse may be seen on television almost every night, and genuine sexual difficulties are discussed openly, for most people sex is an essentially private matter involving 'private parts'. To ask for help directly may be difficult and embarrassing. A complaint of pain may be presented to the doctor as a 'visiting card': a means of drawing the doctor's attention to a certain part of the body. The doctor trained in the psychosexual approach, which uses an unstructured interview, can allow the patient to choose the topic for discussion. Then, by observing the patient's demeanour and attitude to examination with great care, clues to the patient's real distress may be picked up.

Pauline, a rather drab, mousy woman of 35 asked for help at a family planning clinic. She had been to her doctor for contraception in the past, but 'didn't like to bother him'. She said she was unable to have intercourse because of pain down below. Perhaps she had an infection? The doctor began by asking questions: How long had she had the pain? Was there a discharge?, and so on, but she noticed Pauline was evasive in her answers. She also noticed that Pauline was sitting on the edge of her chair with her bag clutched firmly in her lap. When she suggested an examination, Pauline said she thought her period might be starting and perhaps she could come back another time. The doctor com-

mented on Pauline's anxiety, both about discussion of
the part of her body and the prospect of examination,
but suggested it might be a good thing to take a look
anyway. Only when Pauline was on the couch with her
knees firmly together and the blanket up to her chin was
she able to tell the doctor that her real reason for coming
was that she had been married 14 years and never been
able to have intercourse – and now she wanted a baby.

In this case the patient knew within herself what the real complaint
was. Sometimes, however, it may be hidden from her conscious
knowledge. In this event the doctor must watch even more carefully for signs of distress in the patient and in the doctor/patient
relationship as evidence of the real cause of the complaint. The
doctor makes observations which are tested out with the patient,
doctor and patient working together until the interpretation seems
to fit.

Mrs M was a young woman who was referred to the
gynaecologist because intercourse was painful. There
were no other symptoms to suggest a physical cause,
and pelvic examination was normal. Before subjecting
the patient to further investigation, the gynaecologist
asked for a psychosexual opinion. The patient accepted
with some enthusiasm.

A pleasant looking woman of 25, Mrs M started by
saying she really did not see how it could be 'in the
mind'. In reply to a direct question, she said the pain had
started soon after her marriage, six months previously.
After a short silence she said, of course it might be
because of her brother, who had abused her as a child.
When asked to say a bit more about that, it turned out
to have consisted of some touching and fondling. The
doctor said, 'You don't seem to have been too upset by
that', and the patient agreed. Another pause, Mrs M's
eyes slowly filled with tears. 'What really did upset me
was the death of my previous boyfriend. His name was
John, the same as my husband.' She wept for a while,
and with little prodding from the doctor spent the rest
of the time talking about the circumstances of his death.

In the next few weeks Mrs M went through an extra-
ordinarily vivid grieving process. Each night she
dreamed of seeing the previous John, running after him,

and, as she finally reached him, he turned round – but it was not him. One night she did reach him. At that moment she woke and, turning to her husband, she told him for the first time of the depths of her previous feelings. He accepted her tears and comforted her.

This story was told at the second interview, when what appeared most important was the fact that Mrs M had been able to share the pain with her husband. The doctor suggested it was difficult to respond sexually when you were hurting inside. The patient agreed she had been rather dry recently. During vaginal examination the doctor was able to demonstrate how muscle spasm could be caused by fear of pain, and the patient was able to accept this interpretation. By the third interview she had no pain and was enjoying love-making.

PHYSICAL SYMPTOMS AS AN EXPRESSION OF EMOTIONAL PAIN

When we are angry we feel 'sore'; a difficult colleague may be 'a pain in the neck'; migraine may be caused by stress, but it is the dilatation of the cerebral arteries that causes the headache. Physical change may be seen and proven, but the cause may still be emotional. Understanding and sharing the emotional pain may allow the patient to verbalize her painful feelings and enable her to relinquish her pain.

Collette had complained of pelvic pain, always with intercourse, and now on other occasions as well since the birth of her only child five years previously. Extensive investigations including a laparotomy had revealed no physical cause. She had been discharged from the hospital, and her GP, weary of Collette's repeated visits to the surgery, thought the psychosexual doctor might be able to help.

Collette was from French Equatorial Africa. Her huge brown eyes were full of sadness; there was an overwhelming feeling of suffering in the room. The doctor, aware of this, asked herself where the suffering was coming from, which seemed out of proportion to the physical pain described. She was aware of her reluctance to examine her patient, feeling that to do so might cause even further pain. As Collette lay on the couch, mute and suffering, the doctor said, 'Why do you suffer like this? Tell me about your pain.' She waited. Collette's eyes filled with tears. The doctor removed her gloves and held her hand. Gradually, in her halting English, Collette told the story of how when her labour pains started her husband left her in hospital and disappeared. For several days no one could find him to tell him of the birth of his son. Collette felt frightened and alone. When her husband reappeared, it was with a nine-year-old boy. He said, 'This is my son from another girl. Now you have a baby you can look after him too.' 'I never knew he had another girl. He says I am the wicked stepmother. Every time I look at him it hurts.'

Doctor and patient shared this pain together, emotional pain which Collette had not expressed through all her five years of investigation. Collette needed no explanation as to why she was hurting inside with her husband. When the doctor examined her she felt no pain.

Collette came once again, brighter and happier. She still felt some pain, but she understood and could cope with it now.

Whereas it may be possible for a patient to accept the pain of suffering and grief, it may be less easy to accept the pain of anger. This may be difficult for the doctor also who, picking up the patient's rage, may be tempted to react rather than to understand. A woman whose mother had died shortly after the birth of her first child was able to accept that her pain was not due to physical damage during delivery but connected with grief at the death of her mother. What was more difficult to accept was not the pain of loss, but of rage that the funeral arrangements had been made without consulting her, and, in her opinion, not in accordance with her mother's wishes. The doctor felt she should be sympathetic with this woman who had lost her mother at such a time, but instead found herself angry at the way she demanded immediate appointments and then failed to turn up. When at the third visit the doctor put these feelings back to the patient, she was able to accept that she did indeed feel angry and this feeling could be causing her to tighten her pelvic muscles and literally shut her husband out. Understanding and accepting the doctor's interpretation produced a dramatic resolution of her problem.

The task of the psychosexual doctor with the patient in pain is to try to understand its cause. Often physical investigations have already been performed and have shown no physical disorder. By listening and observing, and by the continuing process of studying and interpreting the doctor/patient relationship, a psychological reason for the pain may be discovered and the patient helped to accept and come to terms with it. Not always is it possible to explain the reason why painful feelings cause physical pain, and the patient may need help to accept this too. Sharing the understanding of a patient's pain, often difficult for doctor as well as patient, may sometimes lead to cure. At other times and in other cases the pain, though understood, persists. Here the old adage, 'cure sometimes, relieve often, and comfort always' is never more true.

14

Adolescent sexuality

Elphis Christopher

SUMMARY

- Psychosexual development in the adolescent
- Cultural aspects
- Teenage pregnancy and motherhood

'To be normal during the adolescent period is itself abnormal.' (A. Freud, 1936)
'The notion of normative adolescent turmoil is purely and simply a myth.' (Weiner, 1989)

What is to be made of the above two statements (quoted by Zylke, 1989), so antithetical to one another? They are intriguing from another aspect as well: separated by time, they come from two different continents, the first from Europe, and the second from America – the birthplace of the 'teenager' and the 'teen phenomenon'.

Before the 1960s, there was no such concept as a teenager in Britain or Europe. People left school at 14 and became pseudo adults. During the 1960s there was greater affluence, increased mobility, a loosening of family ties, and the creation of a special commercial market for young people, who had their own music, style of dress and behaviour. Adults who had grown up in the privation of the Second World War wanted something better for their children, and often indulged them materially. Anxiety soon set in about teenage behaviour, especially sexual behaviour. Teenage music was too loud, their clothes too revealing, and their behaviour too provocative. Drugs and alcohol began to appear on the scene. Shakespeare, 400 years earlier, had noted what a difficult age it was between 16 and 23, 'getting wenches with child, wronging the ancientry, stealing and fighting' (*The Winter's Tale*). The two most famous teenage lovers, Romeo and Juliet, were of course also Shakespeare's creation. Juliet, it must be remembered, was only 14!

Two British studies (Schofield, 1965; Farrell, 1978) carried out ten years apart showed the proportion of young people admitting to sexual experience had risen. By 1978, 51% of single teenagers had had sex by the age of 19, and one girl in eight was likely to have had sexual intercourse before the age of 16. As the pregnancy rates and 'shotgun' marriages began to increase among teenage girls, panic ensued. A large number of committees were formed consisting of concerned adults (teachers, youth workers, clergy) to consider what should be done about young people. Teenagers had become a problem to society; the difficulty faced by these committees and parents was that there was no previous experience to guide them. People wanted to regard themselves as enlightened about the young, and parents were often caught in a dilemma, not wanting to be too strict nor yet too lenient. They often reverted to a third way; trying to reason and to be a 'friend' of their teenage son or daughter – which tended to rebound on them. As a friend it is difficult to lay down rules and maintain boundaries, and an additional problem was not knowing what the rules were. What was acceptable behaviour? How long should your teenager stay out? What about all-night parties? When should sexual activity start? Confusion abounded, which teenagers exploited, playing one adult off against another ('Well, my friend's mum says she can go to an all-night party; why can't I?') The mystery was that adults seemed too shy or too embarrassed to discuss their views with each other.

Most of the committees on adolescent problems felt more education about sex and personal relationships was required, and accordingly produced numerous handbooks and guidelines on what should be taught. The term 'sex education', however, occasioned anxiety. Should all the facts be included, or only selected facts? Others thought sex education was the *cause* of teenage problems, quite ignoring the fact that very few teenagers were given any sex education – apart from the informal kind learned in the school bicycle shed.

In response to the anxiety about the increase in teenage pregnancies, in 1964 the Brook Advisory Clinics were set up to give contraceptive advice and counselling to young people. The Family Planning Association also opened their clinics to the unmarried, and ran special sessions for the young. Such clinics produced much controversy, their critics seeing them as promoting teenage sexual activity and encouraging promiscuity. By law the age for consent to sexual intercourse for a girl is 16, and in the mid-1980s there were court cases about the legality of providing contraceptive advice for these under-age girls without parental consent. It is now legal to give such advice if the girl cannot tell her parents, although advised to do so, and also intends to continue to be sexually active.

Other problems concerning young people have now come to the fore: sexual abuse within the family and its effects upon the young person; the Acquired Immunity Deficiency Syndrome (AIDS), seen at first mainly among homosexuals, but threatening to involve the heterosexual population ever more widely unless sexual behaviour, especially among young people, changes.

PSYCHOSEXUAL DEVELOPMENT IN THE ADOLESCENT

In the third of his three essays on sexuality, Freud (1905) delineated three tasks facing the adolescent: crystallization of sexual identity; the finding of a sexual object; and the bringing together of the two main stems of sexuality – the sexual one and the tender one. Other analysts, notably Erikson (1951) and Blos (1962), have elaborated and expanded on our knowledge of adolescence. For Erikson, adolescence is the time of formation and consolidation of both sexual and work identity. It is also the time of role confusion, uncertainty about sexual identity, and who the adolescent really is. Delinquency and psychotic episodes can occur as the result of role confusion, although Erikson thought if these were diagnosed and treated correctly the outcome could be favourable.

Blos has described adolescence as falling into three phases. The first phase is early adolescence, the period of puberty, lasting around three years, from 11–12 to 14–15; the second phase, mid-adolescence, lasts from 14–15 to 17–18, and is the period of identi-fication and self-realization ('This is what I am'); and, finally, late adolescence, the period of being able to cope, lasts from 17–18 to 19–20. There may be overlaps between these phases, and they may be compressed. For example, the last phase is associated with advanced training for specific roles in society, but for young people who leave school and attempt to earn a living at 16, late adolescence is largely condensed into mid-adolescence. These years are above all a time for transition and change, and as such cannot but be problematic.

The doctor or nurse working in primary care is in a privileged position to enable young people to value their sexuality.

Early adolescence
In early adolescence, children begin to change their behaviour towards their parents: boys of 10 or 11 may become preoccupied with the sexuality of their mothers; girls become more seductive to their fathers. Although interested in the sexuality of their par-ents, they may strenuously deny their parents' ability to have sex ('My parents don't do that sort of thing'). If parents have more children at this time it can be acutely embarrassing for their early adolescents. Separation from parents is beginning in this phase, and 'Leave me alone!' is a common cry.

Puberty is a time of rapid growth, which can lead to feelings of being out of control. With their dramatic growth in height, boys are no longer so sure of their own bodies in space; many become clumsy. Voice changes can be intensely embarrassing. As the penis and testes grow larger, boys become aware of genital excitement, which is felt to be uncontrollable. In order to cope with these changes the boy may withdraw and become secretive. If there is no physical privacy at home, he may seek it in the streets.

Boys naturally masturbate in order to gain control of their sexual urges and to discover their bodies. Those who do not do so may find it more difficult to develop a feeling of genuine self-awareness. During early adolescence boys assess their masculinity primarily in relation to other boys; this is the stage of 'gangs', which give security and a sense of belonging.

For the adolescent girl, breast development and the onset of menstruation is a major psychological hurdle, and the way it is dealt with by the mother can have profound consequences for the girl's attitude towards her body. Negative attitudes expressed by the mother may result in her daughter having 'period problems', and fears or disgust about her body and its supposed weakness and vulnerability. The scene may then be set for later sexual difficulties, so that the girl, lacking confidence in herself sexually, may develop vaginismus or complain of dyspareunia. For some mothers, the onset of their daughter's menstruation is an unforgettable reminder that they are getting older. There is also anxiety about the daughter because she can now become pregnant.

> A mother accompanied her 15-year-old daughter to the young people's clinic, and insisted on being present when the daughter saw the doctor. The mother was bright and chatty, assuring the doctor she was 'trendy' and 'with it', and, as she knew what young people were like nowadays, she wanted her daughter on the Pill. The doctor found herself becoming increasingly irritated, and wondered whether it reflected what the daughter was feeling. She glanced at the girl and noticed how unhappy she looked, with her head hanging down. The doctor said she could see the mother was concerned for her daughter, but perhaps not all teenagers were alike, and her daughter might not need to go on the Pill. The daughter threw the doctor a grateful glance. The doctor, feeling now she was on the right track, and the girl was not having a sexual relationship, went on to say that now that the mother had brought her daughter, she, the daughter, would know where to come when she did need help, which mollified the mother. The daughter returned a year or so later saying she did now have a steady relationship and would like to try the Pill. In the meantime, mother had returned by herself requesting help for menopausal symptoms.

Assessing the real need for contraception in such a situation is always difficult, but can be helped if the doctor makes a point of seeing both the parent and the child individually at some stage in the consultation.

At this early stage of adolescence, girls need to be convinced safely of their femininity by older men who are concerned about them and value them, but who are not interested in their sexuality. A pop star or a teacher may be used as a fantasy hero with whom they can have an idealized love affair to reinforce their feminine feelings. Girls usually also discover masturbation at this time. Both sexes are anxious about being 'normal' and like other teenagers – a feeling which continues through the next phase.

Mid-adolescence

This is perhaps the most difficult stage because it is the time for testing out parental authority, the rules of society, and seeing how far you can go and what you can get away with. The mood swings may be intense, and the adolescent may oscillate between behaving like a child one minute and demanding adult status the next. Parents may become confused and uncertain as to what is required of them, and may feel pushed to the limits as their adolescent attacks their 'sacred cows'. Paradoxically perhaps, getting rid of the limits is not the answer because the teenager, who is in desperation to find the limits, may become involved in even more provocative escapades. Peer-group pressure may become very intense, and the most frequent complaint from parents is about the influence of 'bad company'. Parents have to understand that their adolescent children do not identify with an idealized adult, but with the adults who they observe.

In mid-adolescence there is the first real sense of the future, with questions such as, 'What sort of person am I, and what sort of job do I want to do?' The young person is separating emotionally from the parent and seeking emotional relationships outside the family. This process can often lead to intense conflicts, with the re-surfacing of Oedipal feelings in reverse: the mother who had a close, loving relationship with her son thinks no girl can be good enough, and, for the loving father, every boy is seen as a predator of his daughter. Envy and jealousy can be common feelings in the parents at this stage, and as the adolescents bloom in beauty and vigour they may be feeling their age and worrying about their looks. It can be a time of mid-life crisis, with one or other parent seeking a sexual affair for reassurance. The separation process is painful for parents, when they are no longer the idols of their children. The reasonably compliant child has turned into a moody, argumentative person whose behaviour and attitudes can change with alarming rapidity. For someone trying to help, it is only too easy to be put off by a young person's hostility or blasé approach. If the professional person can accept these are often mechanisms against vulnerability and pain, then the hidden cry for help may be revealed.

An attractive 17-year-old swept into the clinic to get a fresh supply of contraceptive pills. She impressed everyone with her self-assurance and apparent worldly wisdom. The doctor felt old and condescended to as the girl said that, actually, she knew all about sex. Her father, a sociology lecturer, had told her all there was to know; he had given her books and articles, and he was 'really modern'. The doctor found herself disliking this father, who she had never met, intensely; she wondered if her feelings reflected something of the girl's real feelings. The doctor was uncertain as to what to say about this, fearing she might hurt the girl. Instead she said, 'That must have been useful.' 'Oh, yes!' said the girl, 'I could give all my friends the facts of life. I was the school sex educator.' The girl laughed, somewhat bitterly the doctor thought. She decided to take a chance and said, 'I suppose that one of the problems about someone telling you all about something, is that it doesn't leave you much chance to find out anything for yourself.' 'Oh, yes, I have,' riposted the girl. 'I can tell you one thing I've found out: men are no good at it.' 'You don't have much fun, then?' 'No, and they all think they're so wonderful.' 'Like father?' the doctor queried quietly. 'Oh, him!' Suddenly the façade of self-assurance cracked and the girl began to cry. 'You see, he's been having an affair; I only found out recently. I hate what he's doing so I go out and screw those guys, and when they ask me if I've come it really gives me pleasure to tell them that I haven't and that they're no good in bed.' The doctor said, 'It seems as though you're trying to punish your father through those men, but you end up being more hurt yourself. It's awful about your father, but perhaps he and your mother are having difficulties which you don't know about.' 'Oh, I feel he's such a hypocrite!' the girl sobbed. Further meetings with the doctor enabled the girl to stop her promiscuous sexual behaviour, although she was left with the pain of her father's betrayal.

When there has been a feeling of parental rejection and neglect in the past, the adolescent may deliberately use their sexuality to hurt and punish the parents. For example, the young person may choose a partner from a different social class or culture, knowing this will upset the parents; or the adolescent who has had an unsatisfactory relationship with the same-sex parent, may exploit their new found sexual attractiveness to flirt with the opposite-sex parent to hurt the other parent. The Oedipal feelings may manifest themselves in reverse and be acted upon sexually by the opposite-sex parent at this time with the adolescent. This can have disastrous consequences for the whole family. Where these feelings can be sublimated by the parent, they can be positive and affirming for the young person that they are desirable, but with the clear message that no sexual boundaries will be crossed. On the other hand, these feelings may be denied and repressed, which can lead to overt hostility to the developing sexuality of the daughter, who is called a 'slag' or a 'slut' – or to both sexes, who are encouraged covertly to be promiscuous.

A young married woman in her 20s attended a psychosexual clinic complaining of an inability to achieve orgasm. Vaginal examination and discussion about sexual techniques revealed nothing. Her husband was loving, kind, and considerate and she did get aroused but . . . her voice trailed off. The doctor felt nonplussed. The young woman's distress seemed to be out of proportion with what seemed to be happening currently in her life. The doctor made some comment to that effect, and said, 'I wonder what it means to you not having an orgasm?' The young woman did not answer immediately; there appeared to be a struggle going on within her. The doctor waited patiently. Eventually, the young woman said quietly, 'You see, I had an abortion when I was 15. I used to go about with this wild crowd – a bike gang. Looking back, I think it was infatuation, but I thought I really loved this boy, who was the leader. He used to wear those black leather jackets and studs, and I'd have done anything for him. Anyway, I was stupid; I didn't take the Pill or anything, and I didn't think I could get pregnant. When I did, I was terrified. I told my mother . . . and,' she began to cry. 'It was awful. She told my father and he called me a slag and they took me to this clinic, where I had the abortion. I was forbidden ever to see the boy again. You see, he came from a poorer part of the town and my parents are rather

snobbish. It took me a long time to get over it.' 'I wonder
whether you did really get over it?' said the doctor.
There was a fresh burst of tears. 'What was the worst
part?' the doctor asked. 'Well, it was my parents' reaction – my father's especially. You see, he and I used to
be very close when I was little. He was the one I'd tell
my troubles to, then when I started to develop physically
he began to reject me. I couldn't understand what was
going on, so when this boy started to show an interest
in me – well, one thing led to another and I wonder if I
haven't damaged myself in some way.'

The doctor suggested that her father had found the
fact that she was developing into a young woman too
frightening, and seemed to resent losing his little girl
and did not know how to relate to his teenage daughter.
Her interest in the boy was quite normal, but getting
pregnant and the way it was dealt with made her feel
her sexuality was bad. Because of that, she now held
herself back. To fully enjoy herself sexually and have an
orgasm would somehow confirm her parents' view that
she really was a 'slag'. She seemed to accept this and
left thoughtfully. At the next visit she looked happier,
and although she had not had an orgasm, she felt confident that it would 'just happen'. She had told her husband about the abortion and her parents' reactions. He
had, to her delight, been loving and understanding
about it all.

Parents can experience vicarious enjoyment of their teeangers'
sexual behaviour, real or fantasized, if they themselves have not
outgrown their adolescence. Hence the delight some mothers have
in being taken for their daughter's sister, thereby blurring the
generational boundaries. Where parents are too intrusive and
controlling the daughter may run off with a man to prove that her
vagina belongs to her and not to her parents. The adolescent girl
may become promiscuous to escape incestuous involvement which
is either covert or overt. Promiscuity can also result when a girl
feels unloved by her mother. Desperately looking for love, she
uses, or rather abuses, her sexuality to try to obtain it. As the boy
cannot be the longed-for mother, he gets tired of the emotional
demands placed on him and rejects the girl. As this process is
repeated, the girl may set out deliberately to get pregnant. The

baby is then seen as a substitute; someone who will love her as mother should have.

Usually girls at this stage are looking for someone to love, while boys may be looking for sexual experience. However, it would be a mistake to stereotype or generalize. Adolescent boys can be hurt emotionally, and adolescent girls can be curious about sex for its own sake. There can be anxiety in both sexes about whether they will be sexually competent. Boys especially seem to need to prove to their peers that they can and have 'done it' – had sexual intercourse. There appears to be a social class bias here, with working-class boys expected to prove their manhood in this way (Schofield, 1965).

In Western society, where marriages have not been arranged for a long time, the young have to find their own partner in the 'market-place', which can be challenging. The yardstick used to measure the seriousness of a relationship is romantic love – being 'in love' – which largely consists of loving an ideal projected on to someone rather than loving the real person. Of course, it is easy to fall out of love as the ideal changes. This stage should be seen as one of experimentation with relationships. When such relationships become fully sexual, disenchantment can lead to considerable pain and disillusion, giving rise to comments such as, 'Well, I've tried sex – what's the big deal?'

The young people who are fearful, and therefore unattracted by, the opposite sex, may consider themselves to be homosexual, and the confusion of feelings may be very great. They may react by becoming boastful about non-existent heterosexual affairs, or by sublimating their feelings into academic work or sports, or by becoming withdrawn and depressed.

Late adolescence

There is no great physical change at this time. The young person is trying to cope with the complexities of adult reality. If they have had no time for developing relationships before leaving home for the first time, they may feel lonely, isolated, and unable to cope with the freedom. Some young people can go 'wild' in this situation, experimenting with alcohol, drugs, and sex. If the parents are non-academic, there may be anxiety about exceeding the parents' standards; the young person may then spoil his or her chances, failing examinations and dropping out. Alternatively, in an attempt to replace the parents, premature sexual attachment may be made, often resulting in pregnancy.

CULTURAL ASPECTS

The foregoing has been an account of the adolescent in Western society. In other cultures, especially the patriarchal ones such as Asian or Cypriot, different attitudes to adolescent behaviour may prevail. Parents tend to be more protective, virginity is expected in a girl before marriage and marriages may be arranged or semi-arranged. Marriage is indeed more of a family business contract. While it is hoped that love will develop between marital partners, it is not expected at the outset, although couples are not forced to marry if they do not like one another.

Many young people from such cultures accept their parents' viewpoint; others find themselves in conflict, torn between their parents' wishes and their own desires, which have been influenced by the society in which they have grown up. Should such a young person marry outside his or her culture, he or she may face ostracism from their own family. Parents tend to be anxious and fearful about the influence of Western society on their adolescent children.

Although these are generalizations, changes are obviously taking place within such societies. The conflicts provoked may bring the young person and/or family to seek professional guidance.

TEENAGE PREGNANCY AND MOTHERHOOD

Research shows that teenage mothers tend to come from lower socio-economic groups, from large families, broken homes, and tend to be low achievers (Simms and Smith, 1986). For girls who lack self-esteem and who do not know what to do with their lives, motherhood may seem a solution; it can also solve the identity crisis and answer the question, 'Who am I?' The girl may need reassurance about her femininity and fertility. Where sex is felt to be bad, and especially where sexual abuse has occurred, the girl may seek pregnancy to make reparation. The girl who lacks self-esteem is often strongly influenced by friends and her peer group. She may feel the only way to prove to them that she really is sexually desirable is to become pregnant. For girls who feel they have nothing, a baby is something of their own. A very vulnerable group in this respect is the girls who have been in care of the local authority, who may nurture fantasies of creating their own ideal, and idealized, family of which they were deprived. A baby can be used to escape from a difficult or unhappy life or school situation, to establish an identity and role, to obtain and to give love, to establish independence and rights as a separate person, or to test a sexual relationship.

Some teenage girls may become pregnant as a result of ignorance or misinformation, but often it is due to subconscious denial that they are sexual beings, therefore no contraception is sought. Early fertility may be biological bad luck in some girls, allowing pregnancy to occur very early in sexual activity. For some teenage girls the pregnancy may be a cry for help with other problems within the family, the school, the relationship, or the girl herself. Once pregnant, the girl may not want a baby but comes requesting an abortion. If this cry for help is not perceived and the pregnancy is terminated, the girl may become severely depressed or become quickly pregnant again. Therefore, the meaning of the pregnancy, which may be largely unconscious, needs to be understood by the medical team.

Adolescence is a time of change and therefore is potentially troublesome. Most of us go through it more or less satisfactorily, although it is doubtful whether any of us would want to return to it – witness as it is to our awkwardness and embarrassment. For a few of us it can be a very traumatic time with serious consequences in later life. Professionals working with young people can do much to alleviate the stresses and strains, thereby enabling young people to enter the adult world with greater confidence.

REFERENCES

Blos, P. (1962) *On Adolescence: A Psychoanalytic Interpretation*, The Free Press of Glencoe, Inc., New York.
Erikson, E. H. (1951) *Childhood and Society*, Imago Pub. Co. Reprinted by Penguin Books, 1972.
Farrell, C. (1978) *My Mother Said*, Routledge and Kegan Paul, London.
Freud, A. (1936) *The Ego and The Mechanisms of Defence.* (Quoted in Zylke, 1989.)
Freud, S. (1905) *Three Essays on the Theory of Sexuality*, vol. 7, Standard Edition, The Hogarth Press, London, 1953.
Schofield, M. (1965) *The Sexual Behaviour of Young People*, Pelican, Harmondsworth.

Simms, M. and Smith, C. (1986) *Teenage Mothers and Their Partners*, HMSO Research Project, 15.

Weiner, I. (1989) (Quoted in Zylke, 1989.)

Zylke, J. W. (1989) Characterising healthy adolescent development; distinguishing it from possible disturbances. *J. Amer. Med. Assoc.*, 262, 7, 880–1.

15

Middle age

Rosemarie Lincoln

SUMMARY

- The role of HRT
- Symptoms and feelings
- Retirement
- Becoming a widower
- The middle generation or the 'what about me' syndrome
- The end of fertility and parenting
- The role of the doctor

When I am an old woman I shall wear purple
With a red hat which doesn't go and doesn't suit me
And I shall spend my pension on brandy and summer
    gloves
And satin sandals, and say we've no money for butter.
I shall sit down on the pavement when I am tired
And gobble up samples in shops and press alarm bells
And run my stick along the public railings
And make up for the sobriety of my youth

                                    Jenny Joseph

Many people look forward to casting off the inhibitions and conformity of youth and enjoying the freedom of middle age. Some may cherish the idea that drugs can be developed that will delay the ageing process. Since the advent of hormone replacement therapy (HRT), such an idea is not so farfetched, but those who are hoping that some day deep-freeze techniques will enable them to be thawed out hundreds of years from now, are living in a world of fantasy. For most of us there is a need to accept and live with the changes brought about by the passing of the years.

Anxiety and depression about the ageing process are common. People feel a loss of energy, concentration, and memory, and may have gloomy thoughts. Sexuality is often affected, both by physical changes and in response to the emotional climate. Although these effects are seen in both men and women, there appears to be a greater and more dramatic change in the endocrine system of women than of men. The hormonal effects of the climacteric add to the emotional stresses of middle age and can precipitate a great loss of serenity.

THE ROLE OF HRT

It is now well recognized that the diminution of circulating hormones due to ovarian failure can be remedied by the administration of exogenous hormones, using a variety of different routes into the body. The dramatic results produced by such physical treatment, however, may mask the importance of psychosexual problems that can occur in middle life. Knowing the power of the drugs at his disposal the doctor may be tempted to ignore the emotional side, attributing all of the woman's symptoms to physical causes. Mary (p. 93) was such a patient. On the other hand, it is perhaps fortunate for women that the physical symptoms resulting from hormonal changes may bring them to the doctor, when the consultation can be used in a therapeutic way – provided the distress signals are picked up by the doctor so that shared understanding can result.

The beneficial effects of HRT are well known, and include the restoration of vaginal and urethral mucous membrane moistness and flexibility, and stabilization of the body's heat regulating mechanism, with the relief of hot flushes and night sweats. The freedom from such symptoms, together with the restoration of a normal sleep pattern, can transform the patient's life, both socially and at work. Often too the patient will report to the doctor that her concentration and memory have improved, as well as her energy and her feeling of well-being. HRT is almost magical in its effects on many women, but it is not the giver of eternal life, nor a panacea for all ills which occur in the middle years. The doctor and the patient need to have realistic hopes of what it can achieve.

SYMPTOMS AND FEELINGS

During the medical consultation the doctor will hear phrases such as, 'I feel so bloated around the middle, and although I don't eat any more than previously, I have an awful struggle to keep my weight down. I hate it!' 'My chin seems to be getting so hairy, whereas everywhere else on my body my hair is getting so sparse.' Although people accept the need for glasses as an aid to presby-opia without too much distress, dental extractions or the wearing of dentures presents great difficulties; the thought of being tooth-less in bed is demoralizing.

Rarely spoken about with the doctor are the social difficulties which ageing or hearing loss may bring. The men, as well as being conscious of a sagging paunch and receding hair, will complain that 'people mumble nowadays'. At social gatherings men may find the women's voices particularly difficult to hear, and the women may become irritated at having to shout. Noisy social occasions are a disaster.

The sexual difficulties may be presented directly, with a com-ment such as, 'I don't feel like sex any more; I feel so old and unattractive.' The temptation for the doctor in these circumstances is to reassure the woman that she still looks attractive, and that her figure is still quite good. This is therapeutically useless, because the woman does not feel that way, and further communi-cation about her feelings is thus silenced by the doctor's reaction. The woman needs empathy from the doctor, not reassurance.

What should the doctor say? The topic should be explored further by a remark such as, 'It seems as though getting older has particular difficulties for you.' The response to this neutral kind of comment might indicate the areas of particular anxiety, such as, 'My husband has always fancied slim, young women.' Or, 'Well, of course, my mother had a bad depression at "the change".' There is then an opportunity to examine these fears openly, which often helps to dispel their powerful effect on the emotional equilibrium of the woman.

The man too is at the crossroads of his life, and may seek reassurance that the virile young man he used to be is still alive and well beneath the grey or balding hair. Buying a fast sports car, wearing trendy clothes, or having an affair with a younger woman may all symbolize the man's dilemma. Fears of ill health, retirement, and financial restriction have to be coped with at the same time as the defeats and disappointments which may have occurred along the way in life.

Present reality may be painful when compared with the original expectations and high hopes. Very few will consult their doctors about their feelings; the masculine defences are too strong, but they may come with a physical problem or with a sexual complaint that they hope can be cured by physical treatment.

RETIREMENT

The change of life that retirement brings may produce difficulties in men who give up an executive or managerial role and feel a loss of status and purpose. Feeling less potent may affect their sexual life; it is said that a man's erection is as powerful as he feels himself to be. Because of the change within the man, as well as the changed circumstances whereby he is able to spend more time with his wife, retirement may also bring a change in the balance of the marriage.

George went to his GP complaining of impotence, which had gradually become worse during the last ten years. He did not think it was 'fair on his wife'. He knew that nowadays treatment was available for this problem, and he was thinking in terms of injections or drugs. The doctor discussed with him how his life might have changed during the last ten years. George was very relaxed and charming, and told how he had retired ten years before from a job as marketing manager for a large firm. He had taken early retirement because he found the high pressure of the job increasingly stressful. He emphasized that he was very happily married, and had been for 40 years. They had moved into the country when he retired, and he had found the days very busy, with voluntary work, gardening, and driving his wife to her Woman's Institute and political meetings.

In the middle of this story of contentment and fulfilment George casually mentioned that he had given up sailing, which had been his favourite sport, because he did not have time nowadays. His friend had wanted him to go on a weekend sailing trip, but of course his wife would not like that. He said he preferred a peaceful life, and went on to expand this by saying that despite his wife's interests in politics, they were never mentioned in the house. He chose withdrawal rather than confrontation, and said, 'There's no point in fighting battles you know you can't win.'

George clearly had a need to please his wife. Since his retirement he had abdicated from having a job or rights of his own and had become his wife's chauffeur and handyman. His anger about the change in his role was so well defended that it was almost impossible to make it acceptable to him and to relate it to his sexual withdrawal. He hid behind his request for physical medication, and it became clear that he did not really want to change, except to please his wife. He seemed to want the doctor to say that impotence was due to his age, so that he could avoid having to recognize the impotence in his marriage.

It is interesting that the relationship between the female doctor and patient in the consultation mirrored those in the rest of George's life: he was compliant and charming, and always showed concern for the doctor's state of health.

BECOMING A WIDOWER

The death of a well-loved and long-term partner can cause sexual problems as the result of the bereavement. When this occurs in a middle-aged man it may cause a confusion in the diagnosis between the effects of ageing and mourning.

Arthur was a dapper 70-year-old man who was wearing a cravat and had sparkling eyes. He told the doctor he had been made a widower 18 months before, after a long happy marriage and after nursing his wife during a protracted terminal illness. He had recently met a 46-year-old woman of whom he had become very fond, but to his distress he found he was impotent. The doctor asked him if he thought this was anything to do with his age, whereupon Arthur said firmly, 'I swim and I walk and I do my garden, and so I see no reason why I shouldn't make love.'

During the consultation it became clear that mourning for his wife was not complete, and the attempts at intercourse had been in the marital bed. Arthur quickly developed insight into his difficulty, and returned two weeks later, brisk and cheerful, to say that unfortunately the affair with the girlfriend was over, but he knew everything worked and that he was not impotent. He said, 'I feel all right now, and I shall return to growing my prize orchids.'

THE MIDDLE GENERATION OR THE 'WHAT ABOUT ME' SYNDROME

The middle years of life are usually the time when the role of being the middle generation has to be filled. Children are growing up and leaving home, while at the same time parents are getting older and becoming more dependent. Although the children are becoming more independent they will still have many joys to share with their parents. But at times of crisis, such as divorce, financial or work troubles, or the illness or death of one of their own children, their dependency needs will increase.

Meanwhile, the parents are facing old age, illness, or the loss of a partner, and they need help from the middle generation as well. Providing such help may prove more difficult than rearing the children: the roles have been reversed and earlier conflicts may be awakened by the change in dependence. Psychoanalysis has shown that there is an ambivalence towards the mother when a woman becomes a mother herself because of the guilt of usurping the mother's role (Main, 1989a). Mothering one's mother is not easy, and ageing parents can become excessively dependent and demanding, especially on their daughters. At the other extreme are mothers who are so independent that they cause great anxiety about their safety, and they can prove just as difficult.

Many women who make up this middle generation are working in responsible jobs and running a home as well. There may be a sudden emotional 'burn-out', and a resurgence of their own dependency needs which cannot be fulfilled. This often happens to those women who seem to be the least vulnerable, that is to say, those who have played a very busy, capable, and caring role all their lives, and, because of their apparent capability, their distress is often not diagnosed or treated.

Such patients are often particularly disturbed by what they are experiencing as it is so different from their normal composure. Their partners too do not recognize them as the person they used to be and this puts the relationship out of balance, particularly where the partner has been the more dependent of the two. The kind of symptoms presented to the doctor are tiredness, tearfulness, irritability and an inability to cope with life in the way they did previously. Sometimes the problem is played out in the doctor/patient relationship during a consultation.

> Marjorie, a 53-year-old woman, attended the doctor for an IUD check. She had a rather frosty demeanour, and made a remark about being seen 'at last'. The doctor – instead of defending the situation by giving reasons for the delay – merely remarked, 'You seem to be very angry this morning,' whereupon the patient expressed her annoyance at having to wait for half an hour when she was so busy that she could not spare the time to be 'waiting around'. In response to the doctor's interest and concern, Marjorie soon spilled out her story.
>
> She was the full-time personal secretary to the director of a catering firm who she had to keep organized. She had been divorced for more than ten years, and had brought up two children on her own. One daughter had been difficult to relate to during her adolescence, and the other had had a serious accident and had sustained some cerebral damage. This daughter needed a lot of help, although she was currently living with a boyfriend who was good to her. Marjorie's mother was becoming increasingly blind, but was fiercely independent and also rather demanding.
>
> While checking the threads of the IUD, it seemed an appropriate moment for the doctor to ask about her sexual life. She had a live-in boyfriend, and she said, 'I really give him a rough time these days, and I don't feel at all like having sex. I just feel so tired all the time, and by bedtime I just want to go to sleep. I get so irritable

with him.' The doctor asked whether this man was any emotional support to her, and she replied that it was just the opposite in that he was very dependent upon her.

Tears were not very far away, and the doctor then interpreted to her what he had become aware of during the consultation. He said to her, 'It seems to me there's a little voice inside you saying, "And what about *me*?" ' The tears then fell for several moments, and she said, 'Yes, I do feel like that, but really I shouldn't, because a lot of people are far worse off than I am.' She felt she had no right to complain. The feeling of the need to be cared for had been unconscious, but the doctor was able to make her aware of it — although it was fairly quickly denied.

The shared understanding with the doctor helped Marjorie to have more insight into her feelings and to be more tolerant of herself. Allowing the patient the right to complain is as important as the complaint itself.

THE END OF FERTILITY AND PARENTING

Facing the end of their fertility is a more difficult task for some people than for others. If the family is complete and satisfactory, the freedom from the need for contraception and from menstruation may be welcomed. Couples who have never been able to have children, however, may find this a particularly difficult time. Although they will have grieved earlier in their lives, there may be a recurrence of that mourning at the time of the menopause or hysterectomy, when childlessness has to be accepted as final. The grief includes an acknowledgement of the fact that there will be no grandchildren.

John and Mary, both in their late 40s, approached their doctor because they were experiencing severe difficulties in their marriage. After 20 years of marriage, Mary decided she was angry enough with her husband not to want to live with him any more, and they separated on a temporary basis. Eight weeks later, she desperately asked him to return as she had had an exciting but disastrous love affair.

Mary's increasing discontent with her marriage had started at the time of her rather unexpected hysterectomy two years earlier. She was referred to the consultant with fairly minor gynaecological symptoms, which, although no malignancy was found, resulted in the decision to remove her uterus. She said she had made a very slow recovery, and had been tearful and irritable with her husband, and not able to go back to work as soon as she had hoped. She wondered why the hysterectomy had been done, and resented the speedy decision to do so.

During a separate interview with Mary, the doctor tentatively explored her feelings about fertility. She had been adamantly opposed to having children, whereas her husband would have very much liked to have had them. She had always known that the disagreement created a serious conflict between them, and that it may have contributed to the fact that their sexual relationship had never been very rewarding. At the time of the hysterectomy she felt depressed and guilty about having deprived her husband in this way. These feelings were shown by her anger against the gynaecologist and her rejection of her husband. She escaped into a very unsuitable relationship. Mary was able to consider and to understand her self-destructive behaviour, but was still uncertain whether she wanted the marriage to continue. She was also helped by hormone replacement therapy, which cured her hormonally related symptoms, which had been overlooked because the menopause was disguised by the hysterectomy.

Women who have had mothering as their most rewarding role in life find it difficult when the children become independent and leave home. Husband and wife may have related mainly through their children, and are now faced only with each other. Parents start off with high hopes and expectations of their children, and it is almost inevitable that some of these hopes will be disappointed. If their feelings of self-value are overly dependent on the success of their children, one or both of the parents may feel dejected. Such feelings can be worse if there is unconscious envy of the blossoming generation who have everything in front of them.

Mothers may relinquish their own sexuality when their daughters are involved in sexual relationships; anxieties about possible promiscuity give another cause for loss of libido in the parent. The implications of an abnormal cervical smear in her daughter can also affect the mother. Depressive feelings about these things can interfere with the joy of the parents' sexual communication and pleasure, and the doctor needs to be aware of the possible presence of such underlying emotions, and to listen carefully so they can be expressed.

THE ROLE OF THE DOCTOR

Questions asked may not be the right ones; questions bring answers which may not be true. Practical solutions to the problems are inadequate and are often impossible. During the consultation, if allowed to do so, the patient will express the feelings underlying the overt psychosomatic symptoms. The doctor has to be aware of his defences against his own pain (Main, 1989b) and helplessness in this situation, which may make him resort to reassurance. Expressions of encouragement to the effect that, for instance, things will look much brighter when the warmer weather comes, are counter-productive. Such reassurance is useless because it merely gives the message to the patient that the doctor does not wish to hear any more about the problem; he cannot stand feeling helpless, and so he closes the topic.

A more useful technique is for the doctor and the patient to be able to lower their defences enough to explore the painful areas together. Conscious awareness is more tolerable than unconscious despair. The use of the doctor/patient relationship can be employed as a therapeutic tool. When the symptoms are appropriate, oestrogen replacement therapy can give enormous benefit, but this is certainly not all that the doctor has to offer.

REFERENCES

Main, T. (1989a) A fragment of mothering, in *The Ailment and Other Psychoanalytic Essays*, Free Association Books, London.
Main, T. (1989b) Some medical defences, in *The Ailment and Other Psychoanalytic Essays*, Free Association Books, London.

16

Intimacy and terminal care

Judy Gilley

A search of the literature on terminal illness shows it to be singu-
larly lacking in references to sexuality and its implications for
terminal care. In this chapter 'sexuality' is used in its broadest
sense, that is, the capacity of the individual to link emotional
needs with physical intimacy – the ability to give and receive
physical intimacy at all levels, from the simplest to the most
profound.

The doctor visiting a dying patient needs to be listening for the
patient's expectations of that visit: Is the visit needed to show
friends and relations that the situation is deteriorating and more
help is needed? Is the doctor required for a limited 'clinical'
function to alleviate symptoms, for example, to prescribe medication? Is this a 'crisis visit' for a new symptom or overwhelming
'panic' in the face of the unknown? Is the doctor called as a
'technician' to effect already formulated wishes (appropriately or
inappropriately formulated), for example 'We want you to get
him into hospital'?

Or is this the opportunity for 'serious doctoring', for active joint
exploration of a significant aspect of the management of the dying

Source: Gilley, J. (1988) (*J. Roy. Coll. Gen. Prac.* [*Br. J. Gen. Prac.*],
38, 121–2).

person? May this be the time to recognize the patient's spoken and covert wishes about intimacy and to translate these into relevant arrangements for terminal care? Not all of us wish to die at home with the potential for intimacy this may imply; the need of some people to die in the splendid isolation of a teaching hospital bed as a last event in a lifetime's avoidance of intimacy should be respected.

> Mr B was a man in his early 60s, a retired jeweller, careful and fastidious. He and his wife did much charitable work. They were cautious, tidy people, and their home reflected this. There were two neatly folded, well-separated, single beds, which had been separate, one suspected, for a long time. They were childless. She described him as Mr B to me. I felt there had long since ceased to be much warmth or physicality between them. He had been a smoker and a 'shadow' was discovered on a chest X-ray. There was no evidence of distant spread, no local symptoms, but Mr B was overwhelmed by anxiety and despair. He became housebound overnight. I visited frequently. He wanted to sit for long periods, although he had no specific complaints of weakness or lethargy. There was discussion of the chair he wished to use. It was a reclining garden chair. It did not match the decor. Mrs B was unhappy about its appearance and made this perfectly clear.
>
> One morning the district nurse phoned in panic; Mr B was suddenly in terrible pain. His screams could be heard in the background. I rushed from surgery, anxiously rehearsing the potential problems. Mr B was in a state of acute fear. With talking, soothing and physical touch his screams diminished. There was no physical source of the pain. He started to talk in a precise, urgent tone. He knew he could not manage at home; he wanted to go into a hospice, where he wished to die quickly. I contemplated the potential difficulties of obtaining hospice care for a man without nursing needs.
>
> At the door I talked to his wife. How many important conversations take place with one hand on the door knob; some pains seem to be unbearable in a closed room without the possibility of escape. Mrs B implored, 'You must do something, doctor. We can pay.' A few

tears, and then, 'doctor, you have no idea of the liberties that man is taking with me . . . the things he wants me to do for him. . .' There was a long silence in which I encouraged her to verbalize those 'liberties'. In those fraught moments, I was aware of what Casement refers to as 'the creative tension of binocular vision' (Casement, 1985), that is, holding together knowing and not knowing; following with one eye those aspects of the patient about which one does not know and keeping the other eye on whatever one feels one does know. I suspected we were talking about physical intimacy, but did not know what these 'liberties' were for them. Finally, she spoke with a mixture of resignation and shame, 'Doctor, he asks me to brush his hair for him. . .'

I was moved to tears for this fearful man, who was seeking some contact and knew the impossibility of achieving it. I realized there could be no comfort, no intimacy for him in dying at home. Perhaps he could find nurture in a hospice. He was admitted and died within weeks.

The cold, formal atmosphere of the house seemed to reflect the lack of intimacy in this marriage. Doctors trained in psychosexual medicine have commented on how women patients with sexual problems frequently use language about house and home as symbolic of their feelings about the vagina and their sexuality (Tunnadine, 1970). Perhaps Mrs B's resistance to her husband's wish for a chair which did not fit the decor, the reclining chair in which he could be at his ease, symbolized her fear of being manoeuvred into unaccustomed intimacy.

Mr B's screaming was potent 'communication by impact', stirring up feelings in the doctor which could not be communicated by words. His screams were for more than his dying, they were for dying without a wife able to brush his hair.

Mr C was 50 years old and had endured widespread carcinoma for two years, kept at bay but then suddenly recurring with a vengeance. He deteriorated rapidly. This was also a childless couple, but not by choice. Mr C was installed in the living room, the centre of every comfort, with the television specially raised, flowers, cats on the bed, wife knitting by his bedside.

She was actively involved in his care. When I visited there was an immediate welcome, their dark approach road always carefully lit at night. Mr C was able to accept her ministrations and she respected and cared for his fading body with the same robust love I suspect she had given it in health. Towards the end he needed a catheter. As she manoeuvred this tenderly on one occasion, there was a shared spark between them of old, happier touchings. 'Watch it, girl' he said, and they laughed together. She and I sat and talked when he was too weak to talk any longer. There was an intimacy and mutual respect in the relationship between this couple and those who were members of the 'caring team' which reflected their own intimacy.

The day he died I spent an hour sitting with her. It was a thundery day, the net curtains blew and it grew dark early. We sat largely in silence – I quote Elizabeth Kübler-Ross: 'At the end, those who have the strength and love to sit with a dying patient in the silence that goes beyond words will know this moment is neither frightening or painful' (Kübler-Ross, 1969). Sometimes it was difficult to feel if he was breathing. She washed his lips tenderly with glycerine – he died quietly. There remains an intimacy and respect between Mrs C and myself to do with those last shared acts. If we extrapolate from the symbolism of this home we see its warmth adapted to his needs, moulded around him with love, as no doubt this woman could mould herself in her lovemaking.

Mr D was a retired accountant, his wife a retired banker; both were 75 years old. Their home was tidy and utilitarian. A daughter lived abroad and visited infrequently. Many years previously Mrs D had confided that she felt it a miracle that this daughter had been conceived because Mr D was 'so disinterested in all that'. For years they had taken separate holidays, had separate living rooms, interests and bedrooms. I found Mrs D difficult – she was dogmatic, with precise likes and dislikes about her doctors. She demanded 'special treatment' and it would take a brave soul to deny her special status. She would imperiously dismiss a partner who visited in my absence with a curt reprimand. However, she made it clear her wish to have me as doctor was not to do with any special perceived merit. A visit usually contained an element of confrontation. She had alienated many and had few friends.

Mrs D developed an insidious malignancy, which was well spread before it was recognized. She returned home after major palliative surgery. It was unusual to be in the same room as them both. As we talked he wiped his eyes furtively. I was surprised at his tears and his protectiveness and wondered if he was able to show his feelings more, now that he was the 'strong' one — mobile and well. He learned to steam fish. She remained angry, demanding.

One day, he asked me into 'his' living room. With tears he said 'She can't cope.' He described her exhausted progress up the stairs the previous evening. He appeared overcome with embarrassment. 'It was so terrible . . . she couldn't undress herself . . . it was so humiliating for her . . . I had to help her undress. Not completely of course', he hastily assured me. Years of humiliation and defeat seemed to hang in the air. 'Please get her into hospital.'

She wanted the teaching hospital and her eminent surgeon: 'He must be a great man because all the nurses are terrified of him.' She died slowly, in splendid isolation, resented and argued over by the surgeons as she occupied space for longer than anticipated.

Mr and Mrs E were a couple in their 70s. Mr E was a retired consultant engineer. Their son had died in infancy. The flat had a faded glamour, with much gilt and pink lampshades. Even as Mrs E became very ill with metastatic carcinoma they struggled on entertaining friends, having bridge parties. As he nursed her, supported by the district nursing team, his arthritis worsened and numerous visits were required for their physical problems. She was very uncomplaining. Her eyes always turned to him for comfort. He gave it and wept later in the kitchen. There was an intimacy in the flat, the curtains were usually closed even by day, the warm lights on in the bedroom, the nursing dressings and paraphernalia kept hidden. The outside world seemed far away.

Help was accepted from doctors and nurses who were then dispatched kindly on their way, but the real business continued within those four walls. I was called in the early hours one cold night. She was near to dying and had been incontinent in their shared bed. Exhausted, he asked me to help change the sheets. As we sorted linen, I shared with him the likelihood that she would die during the night. He knew, 'We've slept together for 50 years. I want one last night with her.' Together we made up the bed with fresh sheets. It was impossible not to think of a bridal bed being prepared. I helped him clean and tidy her. She died in the night. He called me in the morning to certify the death, observed by friends and priest.

In the same way that a good sexual relationship is the private pleasure of a couple, so must the relationship in terminal care be respected as unique to that couple and part of their intimacy.

Winnicott talks of a 'nursing triad' whereby a new mother is emotionally 'held' by a third person while she holds her baby (Winnicott, 1965). One aspect of this emotional holding is to help the mother believe she is capable of being a good enough mother to her baby. Without such holding, there may be disruptions of subsequent mothering, which are made worse for the mother by others taking over and seeming to be better mothers to her baby.

Perhaps something similar happens in the dying situation – a dying triad. The 'carer' needs to be emotionally held during the nurturing of a dying partner. This emotional holding will be the totality of that individual's capacity for loving and intimacy, but can be reinforced during this critical time by external factors – the doctors, nurses, family and others who become involved. But professionals must have a great sensitivity to avoid taking over and being 'better' carers than the real carer.

In conclusion, patients may express their needs for intimacy covertly in the terminal care situation. The doctor needs to listen and learn from the patient. The confessions of the carers – 'This man is taking such liberties'; 'It was so humiliating for her'; 'I want one last night with her' – will be the cues for the organization of appropriate care. The opportunity for the unique individual solution is easily missed, especially if the doctor uses insight borrowed from other cases, however 'similar'.

Death belongs to life as birth does. The walk is in the raising of the foot as in the laying of it down.
From *Stray Birds*, Rabindranath Tagore.

REFERENCES

Casement, P. (1985) *On Learning From the Patient*, Tavistock Publications, London.
Kübler-Ross, E. (1969) *On Death and Dying*, MacMillan, London.
Tunnadine, P. (1970) *Contraception and Sexual Life*, Tavistock Publications, London.
Winnicott, D. W. (1965) *Maturational Processes and the Facilitating Environment*, Hogarth Press, London.

Index